DON'T LET YOUR DOCTOR KILL YOU

HOW TO BEAT PHYSICIAN ARROGANCE, CORPORATE GREED AND A BROKEN SYSTEM

ERIKA SCHWARTZ, MD
with MELISSA JO PELTIER

A POST HILL PRESS BOOK
ISBN: 978-1-68261-307-8
ISBN (eBook): 978-1-61868-863-7

Don't Let Your Doctor Kill You:
How to Beat Physician Arrogance, Corporate Greed
and a Broken System
© 2015 by Erika Schwartz
All Rights Reserved
First Post Hill Hardcover Edition: November 2015

Cover Design by Spiro Designs

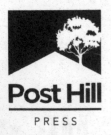

Post Hill Press
http://posthillpress.com

DISCLAIMER:

The information and advice herein is not intended to replace the services of trained health professionals or be a substitute for individual medical advice. You are advised to consult your health professional with regard to matters related to your health, and in particular regarding matters that may require diagnosis or medical attention.

CONTENTS

Introduction   xiii

PROLOGUE

The Perfect Patient   1

CHAPTER 1

The Price of Arrogance   15

CHAPTER 2

The Culture of Disease   41

CHAPTER 3

Welcome to the Medical Industrial Complex   75

CHAPTER 4

One Pill to Save Us All: Part I   113

CHAPTER 5

One Pill to Save Us All: Part II   131

CHAPTER 6

Hospitals Will Make You Sick   153

CHAPTER 7

Solutions: Your Turn to Carry the Ball   181

EPILOGUE

The Empowered Patient   205

Glossary   213

Recommendations for Further Reading   235

Helpful Organizations   239

References and End Notes   241

About the Authors   251

To all the caring doctors who commit their lives to helping people improve their health, these doctors must become the norm.

To all the patients who want to partner with their doctors, this book is a manifesto to empower you to seek and receive the best medical care.

ERIKA SCHWARTZ, MD, WISHES TO THANK:

...the caring and humble doctors who have inspired me and to my patients who trust me. To my husband, Ken Chandler, and to Anthony Ziccardi and Howard Mann, who provided me the support and encouragement to get this book published. To Gene Calderon, my posse of puppies, and my friends Wendy, Velleda, Rhonda, and Carol— you keep me grounded and remind me what matters in a world where it's often too easy to forget.

To Melissa Peltier and Victoria Reggio, thank you for your passion, commitment, and support. Your input in the making of this book is invaluable.

To my daughters Lisa and Katie and their growing brood of children who deserve excellent and kind healthcare.

MELISSA JO PELTIER WISHES TO THANK:

...the many truly caring doctors I've known throughout my life, who've gone above and beyond for me and my family (and some of whom are actually in my family!). As always, I thank my husband, John Gray, who always inspires me to be the best I can be.

Above all, I thank Dr. Erika Schwartz, who is what every doctor should be—a beautiful, passionate, caring human being.

INTRODUCTION

Do you have as much faith in your physician as you did twenty years ago? Do you respect him or her as much as your parents or grandparents respected their doctors? If you have to go into the hospital, do you fear you will come out sicker than when you went in? Is your medicine cabinet full of prescription bottles? Do you spend your days going from one medical test to another? Is the fear of being diagnosed with a deadly disease dominating your life? Does the never-ending stream of conflicting scientific studies that come out almost daily make you wonder if there is anything or anyone in medicine you can trust?

If you answered yes to any of these questions, you are part of a loud yet totally ignored majority.

More and more people are finding that the medical establishment has gone from Health Care to Health Scare, and they want to know how to protect themselves. Many have tried to tame the unruly beast our healthcare system has become, yet nothing seems to improve the mess. I am just one doctor who has been pondering these problems and found sustainable solutions that are working in the world my patients and I have inhabited for decades. That is why I wrote this book.

In 1998, before my first book *Natural Energy* was published by G.P. Putnam, I had written an outline for a book called *Don't Let Your Doctor Kill You*. It was my attempt to raise public awareness of the runaway train our healthcare system was becoming. As I saw it then, medical care was shifting to a focus on disease, and the rapid rise in subspecialties and technological modalities was encouraging this shift. From my perspective it was clear that in order to see real progress we needed to develop an integrated, preventive care medicine model.

The plummeting quality of care I saw was a direct consequence of the trend toward depersonalization and over-specialization that was taking hold of conventional medicine in late twentieth century America. It was crystal clear to me that, with the decline in a solid doctor-patient relationship, things were only going to get worse. I predicted that the system would spin out of control and, tragically, I was right.

My most important insight was that, unless patients took responsibility for their own outcomes, we were heading for a major healthcare crisis. To be able to effectively take responsibility, they needed a physician as a *partner*, not a patriarchal automaton—the model of doctor medical schools were continuously churning out. I could say this because I was trained to be one of those doctors.

I am a conventionally trained and practicing internist subspecializing in critical care, with five years experience as Medical Director of a tertiary academic trauma center north of New York City. Following that, I spent almost two decades in private practice in internal medicine, a branch of medicine that deals with the diagnosis and treatment of diseases that do not require surgery. My patients were a mix of blue collar, educated middle and upper middle class—a representative slice of the American population at large.

Unequivocally, acute care is an essential part of the healthcare system. When trauma happens—broken bones, heart attacks, strokes—acute care does save people who would otherwise statistically have no chance of survival. But once the life is saved, then what? Once you no longer needed acute care, there was no focus on preventive follow-up. The only thing we were trained to do was to find something else wrong and eventually get the patient back into the hospital, back into acute care. Oddly, the goal is to give you medications, tests, biopsies, and procedures, keeping you sick and terrified of missing an illness.

The way I saw it, the demise of primary care and the rise in subspecialties were trends that created even more confusion. I foresaw the new focus on technological advances and the rise in specialization— breaking down of people into individual body parts—as a surefire path to at worst life-threatening mistakes, and at best disjointed care.

I saw communication skills among doctors and between doctors and patients deteriorating in the hospitals in which I worked. Priorities slowly shifted from how the patient was doing with the treatments ordered by a growing parade of subspecialists to how accurately and legally bulletproof the medical record was kept. Departments of quality assurance and compliance grew exponentially in hospitals, while patient advocacy dropped to the bottom of priorities.

I watched doctors stop communicating with their patients. They just wrote their notes and orders, and rarely read what other doctors on the same case did. In the intensive care units there were systems with one physician supervising the entire care of the individual patient. But that was not where most hospitalized patients got their care and, as a result of the lack of coordinating physicians in general medical wards, patient care suffered.

This trend was taking shape in the 1980s and 1990s. At the time, I was working out of both academic and private hospitals and saw little difference in terms of the growing disconnect between doctors and patients. In fact, the competition for patients, cutthroat politics, and behind-the-scenes power struggles between doctors was the same in both milieus.

I became disillusioned with the reality of medicine and sad because medicine is the career of my dreams. I became a physician because I wanted to help people. Politics and competition for money, patients, accolades, or status turned me off. My parents escaped communist Romania and brought me to New York via Rome in the late 1960s. Theirs was a clear message: if I worked hard and delivered the best I could, with kindness and care, I would become a good doctor.

When I started making notes for this book back in the '90s, I was outraged. I was ready to expose the countless careless mistakes I saw on a daily basis. I wanted to sound the alarm that, if this trend continued, we were going to wind up with a disastrous healthcare system that would hurt millions.

But that was not the right time. My agent told me in no uncertain terms to forget about writing this book. It was too controversial. I was too young and inexperienced. She said I was too idealistic and most likely exaggerating a problem that time would solve. So I listened.

Instead of writing *Don't Let Your Doctor Kill You*, I focused on becoming a better doctor. I decided to move away from acute and critical care. I decided not to follow the diseases and labels craze. Instead, I started focusing on the entire patient, doing research that would give me a broader and deeper education of the individual as a whole. I came across the nascent fields of prevention and wellness medicine. In those days, no one had heard of them.

I stopped focusing exclusively on test results when seeing a patient. Instead, I delved into my patients' lives. I listened to their stories and learned to pay close attention to what was said between the lines— how their marriages were going, what was going on in the family and with friends, how their sex life was, what was happening at work, what stressed them and how they dealt with the stressors, what they ate and drank, if they exercised, and if they slept well. Soon, I found myself offering more commonsense advice and fewer prescriptions for medications. Many of my colleagues asked me if I was becoming a psychiatrist. My answer was always, "No, I'm becoming a better doctor."

The outcomes of this shift in focus were transformational. By helping raise my patients' self-awareness, by helping them integrate their lives with their health, my patients began to make connections between their health and lifestyles. Every life is a unique, complex puzzle, and I was helping people find some of their own missing pieces. It was an exciting and inspirational time. As my confidence grew, I watched my patients take more control of their own health and their outcomes were consistently nothing short of miraculous.

To my amazement, this transition hinged on telling the *truth*.

* The truth is that doctors *have no idea* how you feel and will never know how you feel because the doctor does not live inside your body—you do.
* The truth is that to get the correct healthcare for you, you have to understand how you feel and express it in everyday language without fear of being judged. You have to stop using the medical jargon doctors use.
* The truth is you have no real choice but to seek a doctor who listens to you and is going to protect you with sound advice that resonates with you. That doctor must be committed to *you* and work only for *you*. To truly represent you the doctor cannot have other masters—not malpractice fears, pressure from drug companies, insurance companies, equipment companies, or any other "invisible presence" in the examination rooms.
* The truth is that if you don't feel right about a doctor's advice, but accept it out of fear, you are risking your health and potentially your life.

- The truth is that not every doctor is right for you. The doctor-patient relationship isn't different from any other human relationship. If it's a good fit, stay with it. If it's not right and you choose to stay it might kill you.
- The truth is that every word a doctor speaks to a patient has tremendous impact. In medical school, there is no training in sensitivity or how to speak to a patient. If your doctor is not impeccable with his words and care, no matter how adept he is in his field, this deficiency may be devastating to your life and health.

Most doctors have huge egos, which directly impact the outcome of your treatment. I was once no different. I'm still direct and opinionated, but I'm no longer judgmental. During my personal transformation I learned to remove my own ego from every interaction with a patient. I learned to only speak to patients in a respectful, kind, and non-alarmist manner. The result was better outcomes for my patients.

Between 1997 and 2007 I saw patients in my clinical practice and did research in the newly developing field of prevention. I became knowledgeable in diet, exercise, lifestyle, hormones and supplements, and wrote books about my clinical experiences to help people lead healthier lives.

In 2004 I had my own PBS pledge special and, as I became exposed to the media, I began to understand how powerful its impact is on society. I was amazed at the power of the sound bite. I learned to communicate simply and succinctly and eliminated medical jargon from my language. In the process, my mind became clearer and I stopped scaring people with big useless terms.

Today, I have been in clinical practice for nearly forty years and have the experience and the credibility to back up my statements and concerns. It's time for me to dust off my old notes, bring to you the newest research, bring patient stories to light, and write the book I should've written a very long time ago.

The cautionary stories in this book are a mix of cases (I've changed all pertinent details to protect my patients' privacy). Some are stories shared with me by other professionals; others are stories from some who *wanted* me to use their real names. Some of you may find these cases extreme; many of you will recognize yourself in them.

This book tells you the truth and will help you realize your power. It is about how only *you*, the patient, can change the paradigm of health from disease-centered medicine to prevention by affecting that change in your own lives. Change has to come from those of us in the trenches: doctors, who need to come clean and return to caring, and above all, from you, the patient, who needs to banish fear and know that you deserve excellent healthcare in your life.

Thank you for reading.

Erika Schwartz, MD
New York, June 2015

PROLOGUE
THE PERFECT PATIENT

Despite the quiet of the stark white waiting room in Dr. A's office, Ruth can't get comfortable. No matter how hard she tries. She spent a sleepless night fearfully anticipating this appointment. As she counts the passing minutes, she can feel her heart beating so hard it may burst out of her chest. For the past eight months, fifty-two-year-old Ruth has been experiencing shortness of breath, fatigue, and a gnawing lower abdominal ache.

Her journey to Dr. A's waiting room began with an internist (her primary care doctor), who ran blood tests that showed anemia. He thought this could be due to blood loss, so he referred her to Dr. B, a specialist in hematology and oncology. Just hearing the word "oncology" filled Ruth with terror. Everybody knows oncology means cancer, so Ruth assumed that's what she had, though she was too scared to ask. She faithfully made the appointment to see Dr. B, who—over the course of about five weeks—sent her for more blood tests and performed a painful bone marrow biopsy (even though he assured her it wouldn't hurt), but still did not tell her what was wrong with her. He did, however, refer her to Dr. C, a gastroenterologist, for a colonoscopy and further testing to see if the blood loss was possibly from her bowel.

She spent two days drinking a vile-tasting liquid, which explosively emptied her bowels so completely she almost passed out right before the procedure. After Dr. C performed the colonoscopy, Ruth spent the entire week in panic mode because no one called her with the results until Friday. She was told the colonoscopy was "inconclusive," but Ruth suspected that something must have been wrong because Dr. C's next step was to refer her to Dr. A, a gynecological oncologist.

Ruth had been a reasonably healthy woman her entire life, so this experience was the first of its kind. She never missed her annual physicals and pap smears, her yearly mammograms, and anything else her internist recommended. For decades, she had annual flu shots and, when she turned fifty, took pneumonia and shingles shots as well. This is the first time Ruth is really scared. She has no idea what is going on and fears upsetting her doctors by asking stupid questions, so she just follows their instructions. Her symptoms haven't changed, yet no one has said anything about what's wrong with her or what she should do.

When she arrived at Dr. A's office, she filled out the usual forms and questionnaires, signed all the release forms, and handed over her insurance card for the fourth time in so many weeks. After more than two hours of waiting, Ruth is finally escorted into an examination room where she changes into a blue paper gown. Dr. A comes in a few minutes later. Though he isn't particularly friendly, he exudes an air of rushed confidence and expertise, which makes her feel more secure. Acknowledging her only with a nod, he goes to his computer and opens her EMR (electronic medical record). He starts to read and makes a couple of notes in silence for what seems like forever, though only a few minutes pass. Ruth feels so tiny, sitting quietly facing the doctor who is deeply immersed in the computer screen. She clenches her fists and starts to fidget like a little child. She is so nervous sweat is dripping down the back of her neck. The sound of her own breathing is deafening. She's waiting, but she has no idea for what.

"Mrs. Y—"

"It's Mrs. Z," Ruth is embarrassed to have corrected him. It just came out of her mouth before she could think it through.

Dr. A goes on without apologizing. Well-rehearsed and unflappable, he explains, "The MRI you had last week showed you have a fibroid in the wall of the uterus (your womb), which may have been bleeding inside your uterine wall, causing your anemia. You need to have a hysterectomy. Since you already had your children and are in menopause, I will also take out your ovaries to protect you from getting cancer. You don't need them anymore anyway."

"You want to do a hysterectomy?" Ruth whispers. It sounds so extreme. The thought of losing her womb comes as a total shock, but she doesn't have time to process it, as Dr. A continues.

"You are at the age where you are at risk for cancer, and your chances increase every year as you get older. There is an almost ten percent likelihood you may already have cancer so let's get it all out and see where we go from there."

Ruth feels tears welling up in the back of her throat and eyes. But I'm still young, she thinks. She has two grown children and a new grandchild. A few years after her divorce five years ago, she started seeing a widower who is kind and thoughtful and is already becoming part of her family. She's been thinking about retiring from her office job of twenty years and taking up her real passion—garden design—as a second career. Now she is terrified. The doctor just told her she's about to lose it all. What if it is cancer? What happens after the surgery? Radiation, chemotherapy? Her life as she knows it is over. All these thoughts and questions are running through her head at supersonic speed, yet nothing comes out of her mouth. Before she even has a moment to catch her breath the doctor speaks again.

"Fortunately, you're in luck. I have an opening for surgery next week," Dr. A speaks evenly. "Let's just do this right away. You'll need to talk to Sue in the front office and schedule it today, to make sure you don't lose the spot. She'll

tell you everything you need to know. In the meantime, I'm going to prescribe iron, for the anemia, and an anti-inflammatory, to keep you comfortable."

Ruth is speechless. As she leaves the room, tears streaming down her face, she thanks the doctor profusely. For the first time, Dr. A smiles at her warmly and says, "It's going to be fine, honey. Don't you worry, you'll be back to helping with your grandkids in no time."

The receptionist, Sue, seems sympathetic as she schedules Ruth's surgery, reassuring her that Dr. A is the very best and Ruth's insurance will cover mostly everything. She hands Ruth a standard hysterectomy and oophorectomy pre-surgical patient checklist: "How To Prepare for Your Surgery." Ruth can't quite bring the words into focus, but it doesn't really matter since Sue has already picked up the phone and moved onto the next task. Ruth leaves the doctor's office, walks down the long, hollow hallway, and barely finds her car in the parking lot. This is a nightmare. She's having surgery next week... but... it will save her life.

Ruth has always prided herself on being the perfect patient. Even during minor illnesses and the complications of a difficult childbirth with her first son, she never asked questions or complained. She's always followed her doctors' orders to the letter. She was raised to trust doctors, she believes in her heart of hearts that "the doctor knows best." Now that her life is in jeopardy, she feels totally helpless and dependent on Dr. A to save her. As she leaves the building and gets into her car, her mind is trying to figure out what, if anything, she should tell her children and boyfriend.

Ruth's story will resonate with many who have been the "perfect patient" at various times in their lives. *Too many people listen, without a question or complaint, to anyone in a white coat and the "MD" degree after their name.* They accept the doctor's treatment without hesitation. They put up with arrogance and rudeness in doctors who don't even take the time to learn their names. They undergo invasive tests whose purpose and outcomes are never clearly explained. As with Ruth, many have been herded like cattle into surgeries they were convinced were life-saving without a second or third opinion, or even thinking they could consider other options. They never want to upset the doctor and that horrifying stance has led many of these "perfect patients" to complications and terrible outcomes. Worst of all, this blind obedience has enabled our broken healthcare system to thrive.

While many have barely survived and many have died, they never rocked the boat or lost faith in the time-honored tenet of "doctor knows best."

As a doctor myself, I want you to hear this loud and clear: *No doctor knows best.* We may have the education, experience, and expertise—some of us have published papers and given speeches, and have impressive-looking awards and plaques on our walls—but we can never truly know more than you do about what is going on inside YOUR body. Our advice and recommendations are no more than an educated guess that may or may not apply to your situation. Unless you take an active role in your own care, you will always be at the mercy of our educated assumptions.

My goal is to help you never be a perfect patient again. This is your life. You must put yourself first and stop worrying about what the doctor thinks. By the time you finish reading this book, you will have the tools you need to change your role in your healthcare. You will learn to ask questions; reject physician arrogance; and fully understand the potential down sides of every test, procedure, surgery, or treatment your doctor recommends. You will have the strength to refuse being pushed into treatments without being afraid you'll miss a deadly disease. You will go from being a passive observer in your own healthcare to actively being in charge of your life. You will have all the tools to own your care and your interactions with doctors and the system.

I will do my best to give you useful information and tools to help you leave the "perfect patient" behind and become "the empowered patient." The empowered patient is still the same you. It's you owning your life. This way you can easily and fearlessly choose to walk away rather than submit to medical care that doesn't make sense to you. When you allow your decisions to come from fear, you put your life in danger. When you are intimidated by doctors, you set yourself up for bad medical care.

Our broken healthcare system has conditioned us to live in constant fear of a deadly disease going undiagnosed. We are conditioned to believe we must listen to the alarmist bullying of doctors who don't know us or anything specific about our lives. I want to help protect you from becoming a statistic, yet another victim. The tools and information, now yours, that I have gathered over decades of medical practice will enable you to consistently and courageously make choices that are right for you. After all, it's *your* life.

No doctor, system, or company owns your life. Doctors, no matter how well intentioned, can only make recommendations, and the only way to accept those recommendations is if they come from kindness, empathy, and caring—not from arrogance, intimidation, and bullying. It's your body and your life, but the medical establishment doesn't care about you as an individual. Sadly, to the present system you are simply a moneymaking opportunity, one source of income adding up to the billions of dollars that go to hospitals, big pharmaceuticals, insurance, and medical equipment companies, and—though, as an MD I hate to admit this—to some greedy and uncaring doctors. To maintain the hugely profitable industry that healthcare has become in our country, you, the patient, your family and friends—in fact, our entire society—must exist in a perpetual state of terror and dependency in the search for something wrong. Constantly terrified of missing a cancer, a heart problem, diabetes, Lyme disease, fibromyalgia, or parasitic infestation, we miss living our lives. In our panic to avoid dying, we become moneymakers for the ruthless special interest corporations.

In short, you are the fulcrum of a system you have been led to believe you have no control over. Paradoxically, you are simultaneously the most important *and* the most irrelevant member of this system. *The system that revolves AROUND you is not ABOUT you.*

On the other hand, to healthcare professionals who are appalled and deeply saddened by the current situation, you, the patient, are our only reason to be. Not only are you, as a living, breathing human being deserving of compassionate care, you are the only hope to save this deeply flawed healthcare system. Change is a joint responsibility that begins, not just with doctors, medical institutions, or government policy—it begins with *you*. You must become brave enough to demand that healthcare become a customer service industry with you as the jewel in the crown. There's no room for the "perfect patient" anymore.

EMILY'S STORY

The following tragic story of yet another "perfect patient" is told by Victoria Reggio, a patient who encouraged me to write this book, contributed research and her personal stories, and whose mission in life is to help others take ownership of their own health. As you read Vicki's stories throughout this book, I hope you follow her lead—become informed, assertive, outspoken, and fearless. To get there you will experience frustration, disappointment, and anger, but people like Vicki will help you see how making the change will improve your life.

This is her sister Emily's story, in Vicki's loving words:

My sister, Emily, felt the first lump in her breast when she was sixteen. It was 1961 and as a nine-year-old I didn't understand what was happening to my big sister. There was a lot of whispering between my parents and Emily cried a lot. I knew she was going to the hospital and I was getting out of school early to go with my mom to take her there.

Emily didn't seem sick. Nobody used the word cancer, but I knew something was wrong. We shared a bedroom and I had found a page from a magazine on her desk. In the article the line "her breast was removed" was highlighted in bright yellow.

Emily's doctor was affiliated with the leading cancer hospital in the country. The cyst was removed, declared benign, and she returned home the next day. This was the beginning of her journey as an obedient patient. The following forty-six years she remained in the care of this "illustrious" institution. There were many cysts and tumors (some were surgically removed, some were aspirated), many mammograms and biopsies. Emily never once questioned any of her doctors about the procedures she quietly endured. This institution and its doctors could have told her they were going to saw her in half and she would have gone along without question.

My sister was a beautiful, smart woman with a career in banking that gave her tremendous pride. She also took care of mom after dad died. Our family and friends adored her and she had a generous spirit. But when it came to her body and her health, she became a docile child, following the orders of those she was conditioned to believe "knew best." I begged her to ask questions about her treatment, but the idea of potentially contradicting or offending one of these godlike geniuses was terrifying to her. One could say, "She drank the Kool-Aid."

In January 2007, Emily called me at work and told me she had found another lump. This was just eight months after a clean bill of health from her last mammogram. By Valentine's Day, she was diagnosed with Stage IV breast cancer. For the next thirteen months, she had two pericardial windows cut into her chest wall, and endured five different courses of chemotherapy that completely destroyed her body, causing neuropathy (nerve damage, resulting in numbness in the hands and feet) so severe she could barely walk. She also developed a blood clot that left her hospitalized for the last five weeks of her life.

Through it all, Emily was upbeat and docile, the perfect patient. I attended every meeting with her oncologist, who kept assuring her, "You'll be around for years." I still can't understand how an oncologist could speak like this to a terminal patient. I'm not saying that she shouldn't have been hopeful, but with each new chemo drug there should have been more honesty, more transparency about the progression of the disease. Emily should have had the opportunity to say, "Enough! I want some quality time with my loved ones while I'm alive." Emily never asked a single question. She just went along with the prescribed protocols.

Ten days before she died, Emily called me at work. She was in a panic. The social worker at the hospital had told her she was being transferred to a sub-acute rehabilitation facility. In total disbelief, I called the doctor, who assured me that my sister would benefit from rehab. I couldn't believe it. I was flabbergasted. Rehab? At this stage? Emily's lungs had to be drained of fluid twice a day, she couldn't breathe, she couldn't walk, and they were going to discharge her from the hospital and transfer her to rehab?

I suddenly realized what was going on. The bags of medication that hung from her IV pole disappeared. There was nothing more the doctors could do and they did not want her to die there because death is a negative statistic for the hospital. They needed to remove Emily from their hospital, so she didn't ruin their success rate. She had been a faithful follower of this cancer center for more than forty years, but now she had overstayed her welcome.

I wanted someone at the hospital to be honest with me, so four days before Emily died I went to the hospital at 7 a.m. I wanted to be there when the doctors made their rounds. The oncologist leading the rounds called me into the hallway. She told me Emily's condition had deteriorated and that she would probably die within days. When I asked about the transfer she conceded that my sister was too weak to be moved and would have to remain in the hospital and be made as comfortable as possible.

On March 27th, 2008, after thirteen months of torture, my beloved Emily died. The last word she uttered was her doctor's name, perhaps still hoping for her help.

As someone who was trained in and respected the science of medicine and tried to reconcile it with being a healer, I've spent many years questioning how we got here. Many authors before me have written excellent books and articles analyzing our broken system. There is no mystery surrounding the causes of our downfall. While medicine has grown into a huge, trillion-dollar industrial complex, the people involved in its enormous expansion have focused exclusively on technological advances, narrowing the scope of medical specialties, zooming in on minuscule details and losing sight of the whole patient— the human being—his or her quality of life, forgetting it was our job to improve their lives by preventing disease, by protecting them from harm.

The most important and least addressed part of being a doctor is being a healer and caring about your patients. Even the most sophisticated medications, surgeries, genomics, and proteomics fall short when compassion and care are missing. None of us know how long we are here for. None of us can predict the future—no doctor, no actuarial table, no statistics. This is not a philosophical statement; it's the truth. Acting like doctors have these answers is dishonest. In the end, quality of life and quality of care are all that matters.

CHAPTER 1
THE PRICE OF ARROGANCE

"Think: all men make mistakes, but a good man yields when he knows his course is wrong, and repairs the evil. The only crime is pride."

—Sophocles, *Antigone*

"I am the doctor and I am here to save you."

This is exactly what many doctors think of themselves and what they want their patients to believe.

Sadly, it's also what we as patients desperately want to make fact. Most patients look up to the men and women in white coats as close to gods. Every patient wants to believe that his or her doctor, who spent decades absorbing masses of knowledge about the human body, is here to administer their miracle cure.

Nothing could be further from the truth.

The statistics say it all. More than ten years ago, the Institute of Medicine (IOM) declared that as many as 98,000 people die each year needlessly because of medical harm, including hospital-acquired infections. Ten years later, there still aren't any reliable statistics showing that this outrageous number has been lowered, and there aren't any systemic coordinated efforts to reduce the harm done by our fragmented, assembly-line system.[1]

I believe that statistic—terrible as it is—is seriously low, and doesn't honestly represent the devastating damage caused by bad medical care in this country. And I'm not alone in that belief.

17

Consider Tara's story. Like so many of my patients, her *medical nightmares* played out over a lifetime and caused irreparable damage.

TARA'S NIGHTMARE

Tara L. has always had the voice of an angel, but at age thirty-nine—lying in a hospital bed, hooked up to so many tubes, on a respirator—she looks closer to the angels than ever. Her husband James, also a professional opera singer, is singing to her softly between stifled sobs. As she slips in and out of consciousness in the dark hospital room, Tara is barely aware of James's mellifluous tenor voice as he quietly sings an Ave Maria over her nearly lifeless body. Unable to communicate with him, she can feel her life slowly slipping away.

This tragic scene did not happen suddenly. Tara's story unfolded over decades—a long series of traumatic interactions with medical care, one leading to the next, until she almost died. Born into a caring family in Portugal, Tara's family moved to Delaware when she was three. After three episodes of urinary tract infections and four courses of antibiotics by the time she was five, her mother begged the pediatrician to send her to the urologist to find out why she kept having these infections. The urologist examined the child and told her mother that a membrane closed her vagina and also blocked her urethra, causing her the frequent infections. He recommended a minor surgical procedure to open up the area. The parents agreed. Tara had her first surgery at five. The surgeon only removed the part of the membrane that covered her urethra. She doesn't recall much about it except for the chill of the operating room, the painfully bright lights, and being surrounded by frightening men and women wearing strange clothes and masks. The surgery went well and Tara went home. She felt discomfort for weeks after, but the doctor told her mother there was nothing to be done. It was part of the healing process.

For the next few years, Tara seemed fine. The urinary tract infections continued, albeit far less frequently. As a teenager, Tara faced a new problem. She didn't get her period. She had incapacitating cramps and her pediatrician recommended painkillers. Frustrated, her mother took her to a gynecologist who examined her and found the membrane, supposedly "removed" when she was five, covering the opening to her vagina. Tara remembers screaming in pain as the doctor casually tore the vaginal portion of the membrane during the examination. As he told her to relax, Tara realized with horror and shame that he had just taken away her virginity (the membrane was in fact her hymen). Tara comes from a religious family and had planned on keeping her virginity until marriage. The doctor's action left her emotionally scarred for life.

Shortly thereafter she began menstruating, and as the years passed she suffered with heavy periods, painful cramps, and terrible PMS. Traumatized by her early experience, Tara avoided all doctors and medical care. The only doctor she felt ever helped her was a kind therapist who Tara saw for close to five years.

She met James, her future husband, at the music conservatory where they were both studying voice. By the time Tara was twenty-nine, the young couple decided to start a family. After a heartbreaking year of trying— checking for ovulation, following every recommendation on Google, and advice from well-meaning friends —Tara and James decided to seek help from a fertility specialist. An ultrasound revealed a large fibroid in her uterus and some kidney and urinary tract scarring from the old infections. The fertility specialist urged her to have the fibroid removed. She followed the advice. While in the hospital she had a catheter placed in her urethra (routine surgical protocol), which caused her an almost deadly kidney infection that spread to her bloodstream. She required heavy-duty IV antibiotics and was hospitalized for a week.

The urologist recommended more advanced urologic testing, which she initially refused. But when the doctor told her point blank she was going to die the next time she got an infection, she acquiesced—yet the results of multiple tests did not reveal anything that would change the course of her treatment. The urologist told her to take antibiotics after sex, while the gynecologist who removed the fibroid told her to stop taking antibiotics if she wanted to get pregnant. Tara couldn't get out of the hospital fast enough.

A few months later, after Tara missed her period, she took a home pregnancy test that came up positive. She and James were ecstatic. A friend recommended an obstetrician, but the next available opening for a prenatal check up wasn't for another six weeks. The night before her appointment, Tara began experiencing progressively worsening cramps and symptoms of a urinary tract infection. Stoic by nature, she did not want to go to the ER, but her husband urged her to go to rule out the possibility of any connection between the cramping and the pregnancy. Their local ER was an academic trauma center. The triage officer, who was overloaded with serious emergencies, quickly took Tara's history, did a cursory pelvic exam, and ordered a urine test. Tara's pain subsided and when a quick pregnancy test confirmed her pregnancy, the ER doctor sent Tara home with Tylenol and a recommendation to see the obstetrician the following day as scheduled. He never mentioned the results of the urine test and she did not think to ask. When an ER is full of patients with life-threatening injuries, patients like Tara—the walking wounded—get processed as quickly and superficially as possible, sometimes putting their lives in danger.

Within a few hours, Tara's cramps returned with a vengeance. This time she also started to bleed, couldn't urinate, and became dizzy and disoriented. After seeing the chaos in the ER, she felt guilty about taking doctors away from people who really needed help and the ER doctor had found nothing wrong with her before. So she decided to wait for her appointment with the obstetrician the next day.

As the night wore on, Tara's pain increased and the bleeding continued. She even developed a fever. Tara was in agony—nauseous, vomiting, unable to urinate, losing blood, and getting weaker. By morning, she was so weak from the loss of blood and so sick, James just took her back to the ER and called the obstetrician. By the time they got to the ER Tara's body had gone into shock from the loss of blood and the raging infection that had spread from her kidneys to her blood stream. Her blood pressure was dangerously low and she was slipping in and out of consciousness. She was taken to the acute care area. The physician in charge ordered IV fluids and many blood tests. An ultrasound machine was wheeled into the room. The obstetrician was on his way. She was seriously bleeding and in septic shock from a kidney infection, which only thirteen hours earlier that same hospital's emergency room doctor had failed to detect.

Two hours later, Tara was in the operating room. Due to the severe bleeding from the uterus, the obstetrician performed a hysterectomy to save her life. Recovery was long and Tara was in the surgical intensive care unit for a week. Much of the time she drifted in and out of consciousness. She received many units of blood and antibiotics to treat the kidney infection that had spread to her blood stream. To make matters worse, during her long hospital stay, Tara acquired a hospital infection called MRSA (methicillin-resistant Staphylococcus aureus), for which she had to take a drug that cost $3,000 and wasn't covered by insurance. It took six months for Tara to be physically able to return to work.

Emotionally, she may never recover.

To this day, Tara is still reeling from how quickly she went from being pregnant to having no uterus and almost losing her life. James was never able to process what happened or why things escalated the way they did. Even though she can never have children, all that matters is that Tara survived. Tara never went into the healthcare system again.

THE DISEASE OF ARROGANCE

Arrogance—a pervasive and epidemic disease among doctors—kills.

Some politicians like to brag that America has the "best healthcare system in the world," but statistics don't bear that out. A 2013 review article on evidence-based estimates of patient harm associated with hospital care published in *Journal of Patient Safety*[2] states:

> In a sense, it does not matter whether the deaths of 100,000, 200,000 or 400,000 Americans each year are associated with PAEs [preventable adverse events] in hospitals. Any of the estimates demands assertive action on the part of the providers, legislators, and people who will one day become patients. Yet, the action and progress on patient safety is frustratingly slow; however, one must hope that the present, evidence-based estimate of 400,000+ deaths per year will foster an outcry for overdue changes and increased vigilance in medical care to address the problem of harm to patients who come to a hospital seeking only to be healed.

According to a recent *LA Times* investigation[3], health officials confirm an infection outbreak inside one of L.A. County's hospitals once or twice a month, but because of loopholes in the law, the public never learns about these mini epidemics until years after the events.

Peter J. Pronovost, MD, PhD, FCCM, is Senior Vice President for Patient Safety and Quality and Director of the Armstrong Institute for Patient Safety and Quality at Johns Hopkins. For decades, he has been conducting rigorous statistical research on the subject of patient safety. In a peer-reviewed article published July 2010 in *JAMA* (the *Journal of the American Medical Association*) he revealed that each year about 100,000 people die from healthcare-associated infections. Every year, another 44,000 to 98,000 die of other preventable mistakes, and tens of thousands more die from diagnostic errors or failure to receive recommended therapies. Pronovost believes the majority of these errors are indeed preventable, but there's one thing that stands in the way—the extreme arrogance of doctors and the medical community as a whole.

"It's unconscionable that so many people are dying because of these arrogance barriers," says Dr. Pronovost. "You can't have arrogance in a model for accountability."[4]

Dr. Provonost isn't saying anything I am not painfully aware of; rather he is confirming statistics that reflect the reality I have seen first-hand over more than three decades of continuous medical practice—both in and outside hospitals. Glib superiority and arrogance are qualities that are encouraged and oddly rewarded in my profession. Certainly not all doctors are arrogant, and probably only a handful of them started out that way. But we are educated in a system that encourages doctors to believe they are superior to other humans. This system trains them to make life and death decisions in impersonal and emotionally disconnected ways. Medical education takes a curious, intelligent, caring, and idealistic young student through a rigorous indoctrination process. The result is a total disconnect between doctor and patient. Young doctors are trained to follow "evidence-based medicine" protocols and ignore their patients' feelings and opinions (the very essence of humanity) in search of the diagnosis that emerges exclusively from lab reports, test results, and "objective findings" that may have no bearing on the human being in front of them. Tragically, in the world of the Medical Industrial Complex (which is made up of doctors, hospitals, nursing homes, nurses, physician assistants, aides, paramedical personnel, insurance companies, drug manufacturers, hospital supply and equipment companies, real estate and construction businesses, health systems consulting and accounting firms, advertising and marketing companies, media, and banks), most doctors define success by how much money they make, how quickly they can perform a procedure, or how many publications carry their names, rather than by how connected, caring, and profound their relationships with their patients are.

One of the most devastating outcomes of physician arrogance is the lack of transparency, which—as evidenced by the secrecy surrounding hospital mistakes—is a systemic problem that we'll explore in later chapters. But secrecy isn't just confined to institutions. Too often, doctors treat their patients as if information about their own bodies should be shared on a need-to-know basis. They rarely admit when they make mistakes, and do not share crucial information about errors with their colleagues or institutions.[5] All these factors are predictors of disastrous patient outcomes. They also are correctable with educational strategies and change in institutional policies. However, the medical community's need to believe in its own superiority prevents crucial, life-saving reforms from being implemented.

The irony is that reputable scientific research, conducted over the course of decades, has shown that medical outcomes are consistently better when the doctor and patient are connected, listen to, and care about each other.[6] The peer reviewed medical journal, *The Journal of Patient Safety*, is dedicated to the analysis of outcomes in medical care based on relationships between doctor and patients and the ability of doctors to listen.[7]

How many doctors read it? And why are we still doing everything so very wrong?

PHYSICIANS—OR HEARTLESS ROBOTS?

Recently, I flew from New York to Miami to attend the funeral of a famous dermatologist. His name was Fredric Brandt, we were friends for more than a decade, and he was one of the kindest, gentlest souls I imagine knowing. Humble and generous, Dr. Brandt was a doctor who truly cared about his patients. He was larger than life, colorful, and eccentric. He dressed in designer, runway clothes and sang show tunes to his patients. Sadly, the media portrayed him as a caricature because he overdid it with fillers and Botox in his own face. Part of the reason for that stemmed from his desire to test new techniques and products on himself before using them on his patients but then he went too far. He was a true scientist: conscientious, exact, and fastidious. His celebrity patients came from all over the world, not just because he was the best but because he was also very kind. He loved them all and they loved him. I had many conversations with him about his fame and fortune, and it was a double-edged sword for him. I don't think he ever became totally comfortable with such extreme success, regardless of the financial benefits and the fame. He was keenly aware that his success triggered jealousy and competitiveness among his fellow dermatologists, especially those who had similarly high profiles. He was a sensitive man—too sensitive—and whenever he heard whispers that his colleagues were bad-mouthing him behind his back, he took it to heart.

I paid my respects to his friends and co-workers —mingling among dozens of both his famous and not-so-famous patients—when I began to notice many of the dermatologists present. Clad in black, they sang his praises and spoke glowingly of his genius. Oddly, those honoring him were the same people that hurt him by belittling his accomplishments and making fun of his appearance while he was alive. And they were moving in on his grieving patients to boot. It was like watching vultures descend on a carcass. And they all had one trait in common: arrogance.

As my plane back to New York taxied on the runway, I closed my eyes and thought about the differences between my friend and so many other doctors. Fred was kind and generous, he was trusting, and he only sought to do good. When did medicine become akin to big game hunting? When did doctors—who have solemnly sworn to do no harm to patients—become ruthless competitors so consumed with our own aggrandizement, wealth, and fame that we regard patients as just the means to an end? How could doctors who feel and behave this way do no harm?

With a crescendo from the engines, my plane lifted off the ground. Outside my window, I watched as the wispy clouds below us thickened into cushions, until they became so dense that I couldn't see the ground. What happened to medicine, the profession I loved, the career that defined me as a human being? Was there any hope for healing it?

IF YOU CAN'T FIND IT, CREATE IT

In the prime of his life, Mark G. was one of those men Tom Wolfe would call a "Master of the Universe." He held a powerful position managing hundreds of people at an influential financial institution. Stress levels were as high as they come, but so were his paychecks and perks. Recently divorced, Mark was enjoying his single life to the fullest. After hours, he was a wild party guy—up for pretty much anything. He spent his free time hanging out with the twenty- and thirty-somethings he mentored in his business, going on golfing trips, vacationing all over the world, and jetting off to Las Vegas for lost weekends—where, as the saying goes, whatever happens there, stays there.

Then, at age fifty-two, everything fell apart.

It all began when Mark experienced severe chest pains at work.

He was rushed to the ER of the prestigious academic center in New York City where he had donated large sums of money and his cardiologist was a noted professor. Because this center cared for many VIPs—Mark being one—they immediately rushed him to the critical care area. Without skipping a beat he had a full cardiac workup, an extensive blood evaluation, even an ultrafast CT scan to look for plaque. The results came up with nothing conclusive.

Mark was fifty pounds overweight and his eating and drinking habits were matched only by his aversion for prevention and healthy living. He was already on Lipitor to keep his cholesterol levels down and protect him from heart disease; a blood pressure medication, to lower his borderline high blood pressure; an antidepressant, prescribed by a psychiatrist he saw once after his split with his wife (even though it was Mark who had initiated the divorce); and a sleeping pill.

Despite an entirely negative workup, Mark was transferred to the coronary care unit, where he suddenly started to vomit. His vomit had traces of blood (most likely due to the strain, which may have torn some superficial blood vessels in his esophagus), but the team wanted to rule out something more serious. The hospital's top gastroenterologist was called in. Since it was an academic institution, the doctor arrived surrounded by a team of medical students, residents, and fellows. After discussing Mark's case with his team, it was decided that Mark should have an upper endoscopy to determine if the pain and blood tinged vomit were actually from an ulcer or some other serious upper gastrointestinal problem.

A technician wheeled Mark into the endoscopy suite and an upper endoscopy was performed. One of the very rare, yet possible, risks (2-10 percent) of this common procedure is esophageal perforation. Unfortunately, Mark was one of the unlucky few. The endoscopy revealed his stomach was fine—there was no ulcer—but had a potentially deadly complication: a tear in his esophagus, which could possibly kill him. Mark spent two weeks in the hospital, on IV antibiotics, in critical condition for days.

So what caused Mark's original chest pains, the pains that sent him to the cardiac unit in the first place? One sunny afternoon, months later, Mark told the story to his friends in the privacy of his sprawling East Hampton estate. Turns out, on that fateful day, it all started with a very spicy hero sandwich for lunch—something about which no one bothered to ask him when he first arrived at the ER. All he had was a case of heartburn. But, because he was an important man with great health insurance, his doctors subjected him to a series of tests and procedures he did not need. In other words, in their blind pursuit of a diagnosis, the hospital and the doctors who were caring for him, placed an otherwise healthy man in a life-threatening situation.

DOCTORS ARE ONLY HUMAN

Speaking as a doctor myself, I know for a fact that doctors aren't bad people. Most of us are pretty intelligent and chose the difficult and competitive field of medicine for all the right reasons. As medical students we wanted to heal people, we cared about humanity, and we wanted to make the world a better place. Each one of us worked hard to earn the precious MD after our name. Of the more than 750,000 medical school applicants in the U.S. (in 2014), only a few more than 20,000 get accepted.[8] When I was on the admissions committee at one of the medical schools in New York City, I interviewed many prospective medical students. Not one of them told me that he or she wanted to become a doctor to make money, become famous, or work for an insurance company, drug company, or corporatized medical group that only cared about the bottom line. Every single one of them, from the youngest (who was nineteen) to the oldest (who was in her late thirties), wanted one thing only—to help their fellow men and women. They were inquisitive, curious, idealistic, and determined. They honestly wanted to ease pain and eliminate suffering.

So what happens to these idealistic people who wade through impossibly rigorous premed courses in college, then line up to take the punishing Medical College Admission Test (MCAT)?

Once accepted to an American medical school, these promising young men and women enter the process of standardized medical training. Medical school curriculum is homogenized, digested, processed and spews out two tracks. One is largely unchanged from what medical education was fifty years ago and the second is new and shockingly tailored to fit the needs of special interest groups rather than those of patients. In addition, medical education and the hierarchy of doctors who work in medical schools—in both administration and clinical departments—are highly politicized. The politics of medicine will put to shame those of any other industry. Just think about it: these politically driven medical schools are entrusted with the education of future doctors—people who will spend their careers holding patients' lives in their hands. Pretty scary...medical schools treat students like commodities and no one seems to care that these former idealists have been transformed into robots that have lost the very core of what makes a doctor great— their humanity. I'm sad to say that very few new doctors come out of the present system without a significant degree of brainwashing.

Med students are only human, and they are terribly vulnerable. Medical institutions, like all health care, rely heavily on sponsorship from special interest groups: drug companies, medical equipment companies, and (of course) insurance companies. On top of that, state and federal governments strongly influence medical education to suit their agendas. It would be naïve to believe that such heavily subsidized institutions could ever be fortresses of unbiased education or the pursuit of pure science. We cannot expect the medical school assembly lines to produce physicians capable of being open-minded listeners who treat each patient as an individual. Those billion-dollar sponsors aren't investing in medical education for altruistic reasons. They want a return on their investment. At the end of the day, the entire body of information given to and absorbed by medical students is filtered through fifty years of political maneuvering and corruption by special interests.

After four years of medical school and three-to-ten years of grueling postgraduate training in the Medical Industrial Complex, very few doctors emerge clear-headed enough to remember their original reasons for starting down this strenuous path. More often than not, they lose sight of the fact that true success as a physician and healer requires the ability to listen to and care about the patient. Unfortunately, the system doesn't allow time for reflection because—saddled with the weight of massive student debt, indoctrinated and subjugated by fear, railroaded into following protocols and feeling obligated to fit into the medical societies of the specialties they chose—new doctors go directly from training into the trenches of medical practice without time or opportunity to question the grueling process they underwent. Since reflection and self-evaluation at the end of training is non-existent, doctors inevitably become cogs in the wheel of a badly broken system.

THE POWER OF "NOT DOING"

I never doubted I wanted to be a doctor. When I was five, my uncle—who was a successful physician—took me to his research lab to show me tuberculosis bacilli. It may not sound very glamorous, but I fell in love with the smells and the sounds of the lab, the way tiny cells came alive under the lens of the microscope. For the rest of my childhood and adolescence, I never wavered. Not only did I want to be a doctor, but I also was determined to be the best doctor I could be. And I instinctively knew the way to truly help people was to stay connected to the patients.

I went to SUNY-Downstate College of Medicine in Brooklyn, New York and then trained at one of the largest county hospitals in the country—Kings County Hospital. During the eight years I was there, I saw, cared for and treated some of the rarest, most difficult and complexly ill people I would encounter in my entire career as a doctor.

Kings County Hospital Center caters to almost four million of the most underprivileged people in New York City. Its wards are full of people, suffering from diseases other medical students only read about in textbooks. As a result, the training I received was beyond compare. It blended the rare with the usual and gave me a very broad experience base. I was also blessed to have many highly accomplished and unorthodox teachers who showed me how to be a good clinician and an aggressive doctor, as well as listen to my patients and pay attention to clues that might be easily missed.

One of the most important things I learned as a student was the concept of *not doing*. In medicine, most people want the doctor to *just do*: give them an antibiotic, a painkiller, send them for a test, perform an operation that will fix a bone or organ, or cut out the tumor or problem area. At Kings County I learned to respect the human body, rather than attack and mangle it. I learned how important and life preserving it is to stop, wait, and let the body tell you what it needs before attacking. Most important, I learned to take the time to really listen.

THE SPECIALIZATION TREND

My own training was in internal medicine and critical care. In the late 1970s when I was doing my postgraduate studies, internal medicine was considered an intellectual specialty. Internists spent much of their time analyzing disease processes, examining patients, and discussing philosophical arguments on the function of the human body. This was different from surgery, for example, where technical acumen was of highest importance. In medicine, the leaders in the field were doctors who knew how to listen, take an extensive and serious history, and examine patients. The key to success lay in compiling a reliable history from the patient, unlike today where the norm has become to run tests and look for abnormal results. Internal medicine was a good fit for me and, although we did draw gallons of blood from every incoming patient, the importance of getting a thorough, comprehensive history stayed with me long after my training ended. In those days, the trend for doctors to increasingly narrow their focus into specialties and subspecialties was already under way. Since health insurance was not very popular at the time, fledgling doctors were attracted to the specialization path because exciting technological advances held the promise of more accurate and better diagnoses—a perfect match to the exploding growth of the pharmaceutical industry.

I chose not to take that route. I preferred to look at the patient as a whole person, not as an amalgam of infinitesimal parts. I could not separate the heart from the lungs, the kidneys from the brain. I could not understand why the only specialty allowed to delve into the patient's personal life was psychiatry. I believed knowing as much as possible about patients' lives was just logical to good medical care. I loved having the opportunity to understand the entire person and the more I knew about my patients, the better I was at guiding my patients toward more commonsense courses of action fitting their individual situation.

EMERGENCY MEDICINE: AN ADRENALINE RUSH

One aspect of medicine that really excited me was acute care—the adrenaline rush of medicine. I loved saving lives, something that actually happens every day in busy ERs across America. I specialized in critical care and spent years in the emergency room at King's County, stemming the bleeding of gunshot wounds, reviving patients near death from drug overdoses, arresting severe asthma attacks—being in the thick of acute afflictions threatening lives. I loved the ER and for a while my focus as a doctor fit there. As an ER doctor, you never know what is going to come rolling through the door next. You have to be prepared for anything and have a solid base in emergency medicine as well as a cool head to remain calm in highly stressful situations. The best ER doctor is one who doesn't react emotionally in an emergency. That doesn't mean s/he isn't a caring person.

After I finished my training at the age of twenty-eight, I started my professional life as Director of the Emergency Department at Westchester Medical Center in Valhalla, New York. Emergency medicine taught me that—if you pay attention—a very important life lesson emerges from the major trauma experience. Outcome doesn't always correlate with the care we give. Let me explain. In some cases, even if we did everything correctly, following our protocols and providing cutting-edge treatments, the patient still died. At other times, in spite of many mistakes we made, the patient survived to walk out of the hospital and resume his or her life. This revelation led to a crucial shift in me as a doctor and human being. In spite of the doctor's knowledge and experience, there are significant factors beyond our control that affect the patient's outcome. In short, the doctor is not omnipotent. The doctor is simply another human being who is not the final determinant of a patient's outcome.

The ER doctor's emotional life is in constant flux, depending on the type of day you have. The adrenaline rush of saving a life makes you happy and high, just as loss leads to terrible self-doubt. It's both a heady and a humbling experience for a young physician that often leads to fast burnout. But the ER doctor is no different than a surgeon or doctor who works in areas of medicine where life and death often come together. Doctors' identities are tied with the success or failure of the last patient s/he cared for. It's an emotionally tenuous world because the stakes are so high. Unfortunately, there is no support system or training to help us navigate the roller coaster of emotions in the profession. Not one course in medical school or postgraduate training addresses these tremendous stressors or how to deal with them. This huge void in our training may explain why doctors have one of the highest rates of suicide of any profession. In fact, physicians are twice as likely to kill themselves as the general population.[9] As many as four hundred physicians commit suicide every year—that's the equivalent to of an entire medical school graduating class. Depression in the general population is around 15 percent, but in physicians it can reach 25 percent—more than in any other profession.[10]

A SQUARE PEG IN A ROUND HOLE

After five years as Director of Emergency Medicine, Ambulatory Care and Employee Health, at the age of thirty-three, I decided to go into private practice in the field of internal medicine. I wanted to develop a connection with my patients and needed to feel like I was part of a community that wasn't limited to doctors and nurses. While physically leaving the ER was easy, the transition to private practice was not.

Once I opened my practice, I had to get privileges—rights—that would allow me to admit my patients to area hospitals and care for them when they needed hospitalization. The process of obtaining privileges was difficult and I suddenly was exposed to small hospital politics. The medical cliques in the area where I opened my practice hated the fact that I came from the city, was young, and had run the emergency room of the trauma center they considered "their competition." Local hospitals are like small fiefdoms, where doctors belong to cliques and outsiders are only welcomed if they are willing to play by their rules. They want to hold on to as many local patients as possible, sometimes depriving them of more advanced care even though it may be within reach. Most local hospitals don't have the resources available to academic centers. The competition for patients is fierce and, since the survival of any hospital depends on filling its beds, administrators work hard to keep the hospital in business.

The process of getting privileges at a hospital involves lots of red tape. You fill out a form, akin to a resume, the hospital checks your credentials with your medical school and training programs, and verifies your board and license statuses. You also fill out a form requesting specific area of practice privileges. For instance, a cardiologist may ask to be allowed to perform stress tests, angiography, and electrophysiological evaluations; a gastroenterologist may request permission to perform endoscopy, colonoscopy, and ERCP (endoscopic retrograde cholangiopancreatography); a gynecologist will need privileges to perform hysterectomy, oophorectomy, and other surgical procedures. Then you have an interview with the chief of your particular department and possibly an administrator. If everything, including your malpractice insurance, is in order, if the hospital administrator and the head of your department agree you are likely to put lots of patients in the hospital and perform many money making procedures for the hospital, you get your privileges and are allowed to admit your patients to the hospital.

The trauma center I had just left was well funded by the county, state and federal governments and provided highly advanced services, including open heart surgery, organ transplants, high risk obstetrics, and had a neonatal ICU and a burn center. These services require highly technical medical expertise and equipment that local hospitals simply can't afford. Local hospitals are all about keeping their business running, which means keeping patients within their sphere of influence so they don't look elsewhere for care. Remember, doctors are competitive. Unless you are in a referral group or network, where doctors send patients to one another, you are an outsider. No matter how talented or dedicated you are, you won't get patients referred to you because the system is based on politics and money, not what's best for the patient. It's the reality of medicine.

Once doctors go into private practice after training, most of them don't have time to keep up with the most up-to-date developments in their area of medicine. As a result, their knowledge quickly becomes outdated. While that may be fine for common medical and surgical problems, when a patient is in need of acute or specialized care it becomes a larger issue. Unless patients are referred from local hospitals to academic or specialty care centers for rare diseases and conditions requiring true specialists, patients may miss out on optimum care.

After a long process, I finally got privileges at some smaller area hospitals and my practice began to thrive through word of mouth. Having a private practice was an amazing experience. Finally, I had the opportunity to really get to know my patients. I made house calls and asked my patients to share with me as much about their lives, their struggles, and their aspirations as possible. The better I got to know my patients and their circumstances, the clearer it became to me that the body and mind are one and a person's health is directly affected by the interaction between the two. It was fascinating and very rewarding to make the connection between stress and disease. (Unfortunately, this is not what we are taught in medical school and, even today, you'll find some of the most respected physicians in the world scoffing at the idea.)

It became clear to me that, in order to be a good doctor and to realistically help my patients, they had to be comfortable with me. They had to know they could ask me any question or tell me any secret, without fear of judgment. When I sent my patients for tests, they'd tell the technicians they were my "friends" and that reassured me I was on the correct path. In medical school, I'd been taught to keep emotional distance from my patients, that to maintain objectivity, you must be aloof and not become emotionally involved. Providing medical care to family and friends was discouraged. I found these taboos unacceptable and just plain wrong. The closer I was to my patients, the better doctor I became. I loved my patients and they loved me. I went to their weddings and graduations. When they passed away, I attended their funerals and memorials. I became part of their families and communities. And along the way my practice grew beyond my wildest expectations.

After a while, I started having problems with the local hospitals. They didn't like my approach because I didn't focus on hospital care but rather found that keeping the patient in his/her environment worked best for the patients. The administrators took issue with the fact that I wasn't referring enough patients to their specialists or sending them for more tests at their hospitals. In stark contrast to the years I spent in trauma medicine, the patients I was seeing in private practice needed less medical intervention and recovered far better with simple changes like more sleep, exercise, dietary changes, and stress management—the commonsense stuff we never learned in medical school. My style of doctoring didn't sit well with the administrators of the hospitals. They asked me why I admitted so few patients to their hospitals and got angry when I referred my truly sick patients to (what I considered) cutting-edge experts at academic or specialized centers around the country. My peers ostracized me and stopped inviting me to their social gatherings. The hospital administrators threatened to take away my privileges to admit unless I filled more hospital beds. I was tempted to give in, but I couldn't do that to my patients. It just didn't feel right.

One day, I attended a meeting at one of the local hospitals where I had privileges. The topic of discussion was "how to increase patient usage of the hospital." Translation: *how can we fill more beds and make more money for the hospital?* While speaking to about twenty doctors, the head administrator suddenly pointed at me and demanded to know why my numbers were so low when my practice was so popular. Stunned at his attempt to humiliate me in front of my colleagues, I told him that my patients and I preferred treatment at home whenever possible and that my patients fared much better out of the hospital. The room filled with the murmurs from the doctors—some in agreement, others thinking I was out of my mind. The administrator backed down and never addressed me again, but I knew it was time for me to leave. I returned to the city to focus on prevention, integrate commonsense patient-centric medical care with state of the art breakthroughs, and stopped working with hospitals altogether.

TOO MANY HORROR STORIES

"Dr. E, you won't believe what just happened to me," said Emma, a forty-eight-year-old radiantly healthy woman I've been seeing for a decade. "I went to my gynecologist who sent me for a mammogram because the last one I had was two years ago. She told me it was urgent because I could have cancer and not know it. The way she said it really scared me, so I agreed to go. The mammogram showed a small mass the radiologist identified as a benign fibroadenoma, a growth made of benign tissue that she told me was very common. But my gynecologist called me and asked me to see a breast surgeon to have a biopsy to make sure the growth was truly benign. Again, I got scared and went in for the biopsy. Like the radiologist had said, the mass was benign. Am I crazy, or was I put through all that stress for nothing?"

You decide.

A day doesn't go by in my practice that a patient doesn't tell me a personal medical conflict story. My office is in the heart of bustling New York City—one of the most thriving and universally recognized centers of cutting-edge medicine in the world. It is a commonly held theory that poor medical care is limited to small hospitals and older, less up-to-date doctors. Although the previous few pages may have given you that idea, it isn't that cut and dry. Pioneering academic institutions and teaching hospitals can be just as guilty of churning out self-serving, bottom line-driven, assembly line "care" that all too often completely disregards the real needs of the individual patient. In any institution—be it a small-town ER or an award-winning world-acclaimed academic center—the problem stems from the same core source: a deadly disconnect between doctor and patient.

How did this problem begin? Why is modern medicine set up to either kill you or bankrupt you? This book will outline some of the many reasons:

- Doctor training and education.
- Careless assembly-line practices.
- The omnipresent and overpowering influence of insurance,
- medical equipment, and pharmaceutical companies over hospitals, doctors, and patients.
- Financial pressures to perform unnecessary and often dangerous tests and procedures.
- Unsafe and dirty hospitals.
- The average doctor's sense of superiority and the average patient's sense of total helplessness.

Patients are part of the problem too, regressing into fear and childlike behavior when sick and unrealistically believing that the man or woman in the white coat "knows best"—even when their gut is telling them that they're not getting the right care.

Yet, for its all-pervasive, clearly established and continuously confronted dysfunction, we the patients blindly accept this heartless and often harmful system, returning to it time and time again, even after we've been personally damaged by or witnessed others suffer from its misplaced priorities. It's a mystery to me why people aren't up in arms and marching in the streets to demand better care. Perhaps, as patients and consumers, we've been brainwashed into believing that this is the best medical care we can get. Maybe we think we can't ask for or deserve better.

I'm here to tell you that isn't true. We deserve a lot better. My own patients are either contributing to improving the system or leaving it. This book is a prescription for a paradigm shift in health care. Patients can no longer afford to buy into the notion of "doctor knows best," and doctors must bring back a patient-centric approach to healing. Money cannot be the driving force of health care. I'm happy to say that I'm not the only doctor waging this battle against a dysfunctional status quo. There are many physicians—some of whom I've quoted in this book— who, like me, are crying out for change and making a difference.

CHAPTER 2
THE CULTURE OF DISEASE

"It is much more important to know what sort of a patient has a disease than what sort of a disease a patient has."

—William Osler

THE HARD HEART OF DR. G

"*My life was going along fine,*" says seventy-eight-year-old Rosie, a wisp of a woman, barely five feet tall, but with a will of steel. After a lifetime of caring for a husband and kids as well as working in a factory, she is now a widow living in an apartment purchased by her daughter Sandy. "*I've always been pretty active. I go to the senior center with other ladies in the building. It's not the same since my Manny passed, but you have to be with people to keep your mind alert. And I always do my crossword puzzles.*

"*Then one day, the moment I woke up, I looked down and saw my ankles were swollen. I tried to breathe but couldn't seem to get enough air. I have to tell you...I was scared. I never complain, but I called my daughter and she left work to take me to the emergency room. They said I had heart failure! How could this be? I quit smoking thirty years ago!*"

The emergency room was just the beginning. After numerous blood tests, X-rays, questions from nurses, and examinations by physician assistants and an ER doctor, Rosie felt even more short of breath. As a technician who appeared to be no more than eighteen years old started her IV, she was hooked up to a monitor and a little gadget attached to her middle finger to *measure how much oxygen was getting into her blood stream. A thin green tube encircling her head delivered oxygen via two little prongs placed into her nostrils. No one spoke to her or explained what they were doing or why they were doing it. Rosie's shortness of breath increased as her panic rose. She feared this might be the end for her and she started thinking of how much she loved her family and that she wasn't ready to pass on yet.*

After too many tests to count, one of the many doctors who had examined her but rarely identified themselves, told her she needed open heart surgery. Rosie felt numb. Her throat closed with a big lump sitting right inside it blocking her ability to speak. So she just nodded her head in agreement. Her daughter, Sandy, tried to advocate for her, but even she couldn't make heads or tails of the medical jargon or the crazy pace of what was suddenly happening to her mom. Sandy was as surprised as Rosie when she heard the word surgery. She asked one of the many doctors passing through her mother's room who the surgeon would be and how often he performed the procedure she needed (she remembered reading this in a women's magazine about how to choose the right doctor). The answer came right back at her like a frisbee.

"Dr. G, of course. He's our chief of cardiac surgery. He's famous and he's the best."

That ended the entire conversation.

Rosie finally came face to face with Dr. G, an imposing grey-haired man in scrubs who exuded the unmistakable air of a guy who knew he was important. Judging from the deferential behavior of everyone else hovering around him, it was clear he held a godlike position among the hospital staff. His confidence and commanding presence scared Rosie half to death, but also made her perk up and grasp onto a ray of hope that he might be the man to save her life.

"My mother was too scared and intimidated to ask Dr. G any questions. You know, her generation believes doctors are the closest things to God, so you don't question anything they say or do. Even if she'd known where to start or what to ask, she still would have wanted him to approve of her as the perfect,

cooperative patient, so it was best not to make any waves. The doctor never made eye contact with her as he talked. He acted like she wasn't even in the room. I was as scared as my helpless mother laying there with a hundred tubes coming in and out of her little body. I did the only thing I thought possible. I rationalized the entire situation. Everyone at the hospital told us that the surgeon had an excellent reputation. Certainly, he was going to help my mother. How he treated us didn't really matter. I just wanted him to do his job. I wanted him to save my mom."

The day of Rosie's surgery began well. Sandy, her brother, David, and the rest of the family all came to the hospital to be there for their mom. Together, they waved good-bye to Rosie as technicians wheeled her bed toward the OR. The anesthesiologist, a young woman who accompanied Rosie, actually smiled at her and shared some encouraging words with the family. As Rosie's bed disappeared behind the operating room doors, with their ominous "No Entry" signs, her large, extended family gathered in the surgical patients' waiting room. Dr. G didn't come in to see the family before the surgery, but then in the mayhem of activity around Rosie's preparations for the operation they didn't even notice.

At first, the atmosphere was hopeful and relaxed; David brought coffee and donuts from the hospital cafeteria and everyone caught up on family gossip. After a while they realized that no one had remembered to ask how long the surgery would take. When hours passed without word, they began to get frightened. After eight hours in the waiting room, the family delegated Sandy to investigate what was going on.

She approached the nursing station with trepidation and, in a small voice choked with fear, asked if there were any updates on her mother's surgery. The secretary at the desk checked the computer screen and, looking a bit surprised, told her the surgery had been over for more than an hour.

"I was stunned," Sandy said. "Why couldn't Dr. G— or someone—have come out to inform us of our mother's condition?" The rest of the family's

reaction was total disbelief. David said he needed some fresh air and left the waiting room. *Sandy worried that he was going to go out and punch a wall.*

Finally, more than nine hours after Rosie had gone through the "No Entry" operating room doors, Dr. G made an appearance. He announced that the operation was a success. There was a little damage to the heart he couldn't fix, but overall he was pleased with the outcome and was sure he had saved Rosie's heart. Then, without waiting for any questions from the family, he walked away. "Honestly, we were so happy we didn't even care how rude and cold he was," said Sandy. "After all, he had just saved our mom and, at that moment, he could do no wrong."

During Rosie's two weeks in the surgical cardiac intensive care unit, not one single family member ever saw Dr. G again. A revolving cast of doctors and nurses checked on her, but gave Sandy and David very little information—even though there were multiple complications, including a collapsed lung and an infection that almost killed her. Finally, on Rosie's last day in the hospital, Dr. G made an appearance, requesting a family member to meet him at the bedside at 5:00 a.m., the time he usually made his rounds. Sandy was the one to meet him. He told her quickly that everything was "perfect," that Rosie was doing amazingly well, and he was very proud of the surgical outcome. A rushed goodbye ended the conversation and he vanished out the door.

Sandy chased after him down the hall. "I want to thank you for saving my mom's life," she said, her voice cracking. Dr. G turned and looked at her with a blank look. "To my mind, his expression said, 'You don't matter to me. Your mother was just another heart, an organ.' I was left with an empty feeling in my stomach."

Rosie recovered and after a few weeks was discharged to a rehabilitation facility. Six months later she was back home and has been doing wonderfully ever since, but both she and Sandy are sadly relieved they never have to see the cold and haughty Dr. G. again.

The sad contradiction in physicians like Dr. G is that, while they are gifted at their trade, they lack humanity and the most important part of saving a life is the human connection to the patient.

Personality problems exist in all professions. But in a field where we sometimes literally hold a patient's heart in our hands, it's an outrage that medical training neglects to instill the most basic of social skills—empathy. Human beings are not simply a collection of organs. People are wonderful and unique and a little care and compassion will improve not just the spirits of the patient, but the patient's outcome as well. A personal, empathetic approach also leaves both doctor and patient more satisfied and fulfilled. I believe people who become doctors definitely knew and understood their humanity at the beginning of their training. When did we veer away from that truly life-affirming and monumentally important path?

THE GOLDEN AGE OF THE HOUSE CALL

If you are under the age of fifty, your image of a traditional doctor making a house call is probably in grainy black and white; a filmy, flickering picture of a kindly, white-haired old man carrying a black bag, walking up the front steps of a home surrounded by a white picket fence. House calls, to most people, are a quaint, outdated practice that went the way of *The Brady Bunch* or *Father Knows Best*. However, house calls are not an urban legend, nor are they outdated. Before World War II, 40 percent of all doctor visits occurred in the home[11] Doctors carried a black bag, known as a Gladstone bag, and went to the homes of patients who had no transportation or were too ill to get out of bed. Hospitals were few and catered to the poor and those suffering with infectious or terminal illnesses. A trip to a hospital was a last ditch effort to get help. Our great-great-grandparents would never have dreamed of rushing to an ER with a fever or shortness of breath or the flu. Instead, they would somehow get a message to the family doctor. Back then, doctors made house calls for pretty much all medical needs—a woman giving birth, a man having a heart attack, a child with a broken bone, or a flu epidemic. Primary care doctors were known as "General Practitioners" because they had the wide range of knowledge and abilities to perform any type of medical treatment, from taking out an appendix on the kitchen table, to setting bones, delivering babies, and sewing up wounds.

Modern science has given us wonderful tools that doctors who made house calls didn't have—tools for diagnosis and treatment of all types of medical problems. But human beings are made up of more than the numbers on a blood test or the results of an MRI, CT, or PET scan. The house-call doctors of old had a huge advantage that's lost on today's medical professionals: They knew how to listen to their patients and care for them as complete human beings, not just a collection of organs and diseases. They interacted with patients' families and knew the conditions in which they lived. They knew what jobs they had, how much physical activity they got, and what kind of stressors and environmental factors affected them. Because of this level of connection, the family doctor was less likely to be misled by a patient's perception—to underplay a malady, exaggerate a complaint, or overlook contributory problems and issues. As a result, despite their lack of high-tech equipment, doctors during the era of house calls often provided high quality care with limited tools.

Lest you think I'm waxing nostalgic over those long ago simpler days, a number of recent studies on modern-day home-visit-based health care have shown, in both numbers and dollars, that those of us who sing the praises of house calls may actually be on to something. A 2002 international study[12] showed that elderly patients who received home visits showed a 40 percent reduction in rate of hospitalization, 38 percent shorter length of stay when hospitalization was necessary compared with the prior year when they weren't getting home visits, and even a reduction in mortality in younger patients who received house calls. In addition, house-call/home-care doctors were able to identify more new problems based on insights obtained through visiting a patient in his/her own environment and patients reported far more positive experiences with house calls. This study showed more than nine house calls to a patient reduced nursing home admissions, functional decline, and mortality in seniors over a period of more than a year. And, according to one modern day black-bag advocate, Dr. Bruce Leff of Johns Hopkins,[13] "You learn more about the patient in five minutes at home than in five visits to the office." In terms of ambulance costs and ER bills, the savings to insurance, Medicare, and Medicaid—not to mention the overall savings to our society in general—are simply staggering.

BURYING THE BLACK BAG

If house calls are so cost effective and beneficial, why did they vanish? Why did they become "obsolete"? Over the course of healthcare history, interactions between doctors and patients that took place in the patient's home were long lasting, personal and based on trust. However, while in the 1930s house calls made up 40 percent of physician interaction with patients, by 1950 that number dropped to 10 percent, and by 1980 house visits only accounted for 1 percent.[14]

So what happened to the black bag and those carrying it to the patient's home?

Technological advances in the second half of the 20th century changed the face of medicine. The more diagnostic tools and advanced treatments became available in hospitals and clinics, the more patients started to go to hospitals and specialized centers for treatment. Both doctors and patients began associating "good medicine" with modern hospitals, clinics, and diagnostic centers. There were also financial incentives working against house calls. As more doctors specialized and increasingly relied on advanced technologies and specialized testing, primary care medicine became less lucrative. Meanwhile, the growth and expansion of insurance companies, which did not pay for home visits, dis-incentivized doctors from making them. Thus the house call fell out of date.

Finally, in 2015, there is a resurgence in support of the house call, specifically with a movement for Medicare to pay for house calls in hopes of containing skyrocketing healthcare costs for the elderly and handicapped. The results of a revival of house calls could very well spark the desperately needed kind of revolution in medicine that some of us have been advocating for decades. In study after study, modern-day house call doctors report feeling far more fulfilled and happier at their jobs than higher paid doctors in highly technological subspecialties.[15]

A PHILOSOPHICAL SHIFT

As I mentioned before, three significant factors in the demise of the house call and the disappearance of the trusted and beloved family doctor—where the patient-centric model dominated medicine— are the rise in overspecialization, a healthcare system where only the bottom line matters, and the continuous focus on advancing medical technology.

By the mid-1960s, American medical training had undergone a dramatic shift. As a direct outgrowth of rapid advances in technology, the exodus of doctors from primary care to increasingly narrowly specialized fields, America became recognized as the world leader in healthcare innovation. This wasn't just a change of direction; it was a revolution in both the philosophy and practice of medicine. Within a mere three decades, medical advancements like CT, MRI and PET scanning, endoscopy, arthroscopy, cardiac surgery, cardiac stenting, and joint and organ replacement—just to name a few—came to define American health care. To maintain the leadership position, it was essential that doctors become specialists.

In the beginning, specialization in medicine was a positive development. From a statistical perspective, advanced technology and highly trained experts in these cutting edge technologies seemed to save and improve lives. The change in direction ushered in a new era of more disease diagnoses, research and development of innumerable new drugs, tests, procedures and vaccines, and ever-expanding numbers of medical options available to the public that were previously unimaginable. In the process, these developments began to fuel the trillion-dollar industry that health care was to become.

But the shift in medical thinking did not stop there. A sea change in thinking occurred in parallel with technological growth and in-depth specialization, as medical care became a disease-centered business. To satisfy the industry's growing financial needs, more drugs, more testing, and more specialists were created which all needed more diseases to justify their existence.

To give a simplistic example: In an earlier time, if a patient had a fever, the doctor could only see the symptom—the fever. With no immediate tools to identify the cause of the fever, the prescription was often bed rest in the hope that the body would heal itself. Sometimes it did, sometimes it didn't. Today, if a patient has a fever, a doctor will run a battery of tests to determine what is causing the fever. Very seldom will the patient or the doctor wait to see how the patient's body heals itself. This advancement, however, comes with limitations. The more we started to test; the more the testing became standard medical practice and the more it became the only way to practice medicine. If the testing revealed an abnormality, a potential connection for the cause of the fever—a label—diagnosis would be made, and a prescription generated for a particular medication. While hypothetically this is a great idea and we all think it shows we are evolved, there are lots of down sides to the path medical care took. Let's say in the outdated past, a fever was treated with rest. Today, most people treat a fever with over-the-counter medications. If that doesn't work, a visit to a doctor or clinic may lead to blood and urine tests or just an *a priori* prescription for an antibiotic. If the fever still doesn't resolve, an entire slew of diagnostic testing and visits to specialists will most likely follow. The chances of something significant causing the fever are infinitesimal and the aggressive stance on diagnosis is more likely to cause harm than leaving the body to heal by itself.

The enormous amount of testing, instruments, equipment, and processing of laboratory samples requires time, is very expensive, and above all, makes lots of money for the system. While this approach has helped the healthcare industry grow in size and importance, the focus on money is deadly and it has also increasingly led to bad medicine.

To become a doctor, you must commit to memory massive amounts of information covering a large number of advanced scientific subjects: biochemistry, anatomy, pathology, statistics, physiology, genetics, pharmacology, microbiology, and others all of which focus exclusively on detection, diagnosis, and treatment of disease. The most highly respected doctors are experts in "differential diagnosis," the process of identifying and then distinguishing between diseases and conditions presenting with similar symptoms or test results.

An unfortunate side effect of this formulaic equation is that patients become, to the doctor, these diseases. They become a disjointed collection of potentially diseased body parts and organs. The more a doctor is trained to see people this way, the less likely s/he is to see them as human beings. The focus becomes so narrow, it's like Humpty Dumpty on the wall—once the egg shatters it's practically impossible to put the pieces back together again. The patient becomes a series of diseases and conditions, each attended to by different specialists, who rarely (if ever) communicate with one other. Not only have these specialists lost the ability to grasp the concept of the person as a whole, not one of them has the knowledge or training to integrate the pieces. The result is all too often disastrous for the patient.

MONEY AND MEDICINE

The changes that have occurred in the practice of medicine over the past five decades—fueled by an influx of funding sponsored by pharmaceutical, instrument manufacturers, biotech companies, and insurance conglomerates—have traded the house call with the old-time doctor, with his personal, commonsense relationship with the patients, for a very different kind of practice. Who has time to talk to a patient about his/her personal life when the focus has turned to microscopic, genetic testing, and statistical details of a diagnosis? Take, for example, the class of autoimmune diseases, where the body turns against itself. We have diagnostic tests and drug treatments for these diseases, and specialists who focus solely on research, diagnosis, and treatment of these diseases. These specialists will evaluate genetic mutations, abnormality in proteins, and immune factors, yet rarely will s/he consider the possibility that the acute phases of the disease may be triggered by stress, dietary abuse, sedentary lifestyle, or sleep disorders. Without looking at the whole picture, the isolated pieces of a puzzle can never put together a picture that really represents the reality of a human being's life.

To become a general practitioner today, you have to care more about the patient than financial gain, which is often a difficult choice to make. Adding insult to injury, academically-based, overspecialized doctors tend to look down their noses at general practitioners, banishing them to second class citizen status. Similarly, when a patient winds up in the emergency room with an acute problem, ER doctors consistently look down on the care provided by a primary care doctor (PMD, PMP, or LMD). Although ER doctors never get to know the patients like their primary care doctors do, they consistently discard the type of care the patient receives outside the ER.

We live in a financially driven world. Saddled with crushing debt for their medical education that takes decades to pay back, the overwhelmed, overworked medical student will reach for the nearest shiny object in sight. Twinkling just within reach is the promise of the financial windfall a subspecialty may offer. The more testing there is, the more gadgets are necessary to make a diagnosis, the more insurance companies will pay. Student loans will get paid off quickly and life becomes economically stable. It's easy to see the progression from idealistic medical student to callous, financially motivated specialized doctor.

Specialists are necessary, there's no doubt about that. We need doctors with advanced, finely tuned tools and experience—like Dr. G who fixed Rosie's heart—but is it a normal trade off for that type of super-specialist to disregard the human whose heart he is saving? Don't we need both the primary care doctor and the specialist? Wouldn't the outcome be better if they worked together in the patient's service?

THE DISEASE MODEL OF PUBLIC HEALTH

Starting at the dawn of the industrial revolution, from the mid 1700's up to the end of the 19th century, European populations migrated in waves from the countryside to the increasingly economically vibrant industrialized cities. Travelling right alongside them were infectious diseases, which spread rapidly in the overcrowded, unsanitary conditions in which most poor city dwellers lived. During a two-hundred-year period, more than one hundred deadly plague epidemics swept across Europe: the Black Death, cholera, malaria, small pox, measles, typhus, tuberculosis, scarlet fever. Millions of lives were lost. The Americas were hit hard as well. In reaction to the most urgent public health crisis in modern medicine's history, medicine was forced to quickly mature. Medieval superstitions, where disease was blamed on sin or some weakness in the sufferer, evaporated. Once epidemiology rose to make the connection between bacteria, viruses and their modes of transmission, doctors and public health officials began working together to quarantine the sick and figure out how to most efficiently stop epidemic killer diseases in their tracks. The first hospitals came into existence to isolate the contagious and the indigent, and most doctors were trained in medical schools adjacent to these hospitals.

Thus, the model of health care that dominates the delivery and research of all our conventionally sanctioned medical practices to this day was created in the middle of infectious disease epidemics with millions of people dying. It's easy to see, then, why disease and fear of disease were cast in permanent starring roles on the stage of western medicine.

HOW'S YOUR DISEASE TODAY?

Our culture is fascinated with disease. Think about conversations you've had with friends at dinner parties or other social gatherings. How often does the conversation turn to the number of doctor visits you've had lately, the weird symptoms you're experiencing, and the infinite number of tests that have been performed on you? It has become an odd game of one-upmanship as to who's got the more serious illness, undergone the most surgeries, has taken the most tests, or knows more "top" experts. Consider how much more pleasurable (and helpful) it would be if the conversation centered around what we are doing to prevent illness and what methods we are using to teach our children ways to lead lives of wellness and health. Perhaps focusing on enjoying our lives and making them about quality just is not dramatic enough?

It's almost as if disease itself has become sexy. Think about how many of our role models are applauded and see a spike in their popularity when they talk or tweet about their illnesses. How often do you see on television or read in pop culture magazines stories of celebrities bravely revealing their battles with a variety of illnesses: bipolar depression, eating disorders, cancers, infertility—everything you can think of that is disease or disease-related. And when a celebrity comes out with a new book or public confession of a disease, people come out of the woodwork convinced they too have the same disease, for which they run to ERs or doctors who are more than willing to oblige with tests and infinite numbers of treatments.

I don't want to sound callous or uncaring. I applaud many of the celebrities who honestly and in the open face adversity with dignity and courage. Their stories often help raise awareness of diseases that have otherwise been ignored for far too long. But no one is asking the most important question: what are the connections between these diseases and the lifestyles of those who suffer from them? Very few look deep enough for a solution or a thread of hope for preventing the problem in the first place. Our focus begins with the diagnosis of the disease, rarely questioning why these diseases happen to the particular person in the first place. Perhaps, in our culture, all we want is to take possession of disease, to claim ownership of it. I can't even tell you how often I see patients who refer to *my cancer, my arthritis, my diabetes, my high blood pressure*—but not *my health*. I firmly believe the first step toward change is for us to eliminate this personal identification with a particular disease.

IN SEARCH OF A DIAGNOSIS

When I first saw Elsa, she was a fifty-two-year-old single woman who had spent her entire life successfully climbing the corporate ladder. Eventually, though, she got stuck in middle management at a global finance corporation. Time passed too fast and she missed the opportunity to get married or have children. Over time, Elsa found herself lonely, tired, and disappointed by her work and life. As the fatigue lingered and she became stuck in limbo at work, she decided the fatigue was clearly a symptom of an illness and thus began her pilgrimage into the medical world.

After many unsatisfactory visits to her primary care physician, which resulted in innumerable blood tests, CT scans, and MRIs, her doctor decreed he could find nothing wrong with her and recommended she stop the testing, go home and continue her life, and return in six months if she wasn't feeling better.

Elsa did not want to wait. A few months later, in the dead of winter, she found herself suffering from a cold that settled in her chest. After a series of coughing spells that kept her up all night, instead of going back to her primary care doctor who hadn't offered a satisfactory diagnosis for the fatigue, she went directly to a pulmonary specialist. The pulmonologist had Elsa undergo more tests. A chest X-ray showed some infiltrates (pointing to possible bronchitis) and her pulmonary function tests showed her lung capacity was smaller than expected for her age. With bronchitis and bad cough this isn't an unusual finding. Elsa was also a closet smoker, but never told any doctor about it because she knew they would tell her to quit.

After several courses of antibiotics—from which she developed a few yeast infections—lack of sleep from the cough, and the stress, night sweats, and other symptoms of menopause (which had worsened and led to more anxiety), Elsa turned to the Internet for answers. (While "diagnosis by Internet" may be tempting—simply type a collection of symptoms into a web browser and any number of sites will pop up to inform you on your condition or disease—it comes with some seriously dangerous pitfalls.) Elsa became obsessed with reading about lung disease and, convinced her doctors were missing a very serious and deadly illness, she went on disability at work and made an appointment with the head of lung transplant at a prominent New York hospital. This was a huge leap, but Elsa didn't want to waste any time. She knew in her heart of hearts she was sick and no one was helping her. The transplant doctor went over her prior test results in excruciating detail. He assured her she definitely did not need a transplant, yet she insisted on going through an entirely new battery of tests for transplant candidates just to see if there might be a possibility he was wrong. Despite her doctors' advice to wait and see if her body would heal itself in time, Elsa continued to focus on the abnormal lung function tests and her shortness of breath which she felt was worsening with each passing day, regardless of the fact that all her other tests consistently showed there was no real indication for such drastic treatment.

By identifying herself with a disease, Elsa had found a way out of a life in which she was utterly unhappy, yet there was no life beyond the never-ending search for a diagnosis. Elsa's case is not unique. Once in disease-seeking mode, it becomes increasingly difficult to view life through any other lens. *We become obsessed with our disease.*

Elsa came to see me after she had been turned down for a lung transplant. I reviewed the history and data she brought me. I recommended she start by taking better care of herself by improving her diet, kicking her secret smoking habit (which I was able to get her to admit), increasing her physical activity, and starting her on a course of hormones to help her get into better balance. I also recommended she see a therapist to help her deal with the underlying emotional issues that were preventing her from making the most out of the life she had.

Initially, Elsa followed my advice. She took the hormones, drank water rather than vodka and coffee, started walking thirty minutes a day, and took medication and supplements to help her get eight hours of sleep a night. Within a few months she was remarkably better. Her pulmonary tests reflected her improved health and her doctors told her to continue doing whatever it was that she was doing (although, ironically, none of them had the time to talk to me or find out why things had improved). Then, one day, she got a call from work. Her disability was running out and if her health continued to improve, she would have to return to work. The last thing Elsa wanted was to go back to her stale job. She blamed work for the fact that she never had a family and felt it had become a dead end for her.

She made a choice that destroyed her life. She stopped all the treatments with me, went back to smoking, and she eventually found a doctor who would perform the surgery. She had a lung transplant two years later. She spent the next ten years housebound, permanently handicapped, dependent on oxygen, in a wheelchair. She died alone in a nursing home at the age of fifty-eight.

———————————

Elsa's story may be extreme, but it isn't as unusual as you may think. While finding a team of doctors willing to perform an unnecessary lung transplant is rare, it is shocking how many doctors are willing to perform life-altering surgeries just because the patient insists. And, because you can always find a doctor willing to order more tests, prescribe more medications, and perform unnecessary procedures, it is easy to become overly focused on the perceived necessity to fix and find something wrong, rather than take responsibility for our lives and implement the important changes that will ultimately improve our quality of life.

THRIVING ON ILLNESS

Elsa seems like an extreme case, but there are many who manipulate and exploit the weaknesses in our healthcare system in a misguided attempt to "fix" their own unhappy lives. People just like Elsa capitalize on our disease-centered culture and spend their time searching for doctors to validate their often deadly self-diagnosis and fulfill a morbid need to have their lives defined by disease so they become victims rather than responsible adults.

When one doctor did not go along with Elsa's agenda, she went *doctor-shopping*, a term that refers to the practice of going from one doctor to another in search of a doctor willing to agree with the patient's predetermined diagnosis. Most doctor-shoppers don't tell themselves or the doctor the truth. Like Elsa, with her "secret" smoking and drinking, patients intentionally omit significant facts about their lifestyle and habits, either out of shame, fear of having to confront their own demons, or a need to obscure contributing factors that would alter treatment course and outcome. Unfortunately, if you go to enough doctors or healthcare providers, eventually you will find the one who will agree to do something invasive and life altering, even if it's not in the patient's best interest.

The practice of doctor-shopping is harmful not only to the perpetrator, but to our entire healthcare system. One of the obvious outcomes is the skyrocketing costs of medical care. The more tests, procedures and sick people requiring expensive care, the more money the system makes and costs. We could greatly reduce and even eradicate this practice, by simply fostering a culture of prevention and honesty in health care. If we all decided to stop looking for illness and disease and instead focused on making lifestyle choices that promote better health, stories like Elsa's would rapidly become a thing of the past. If doctors were honest and just refused to go along with patients making unreasonable requests, the system would rapidly improve. When Elsa came to see me, I presented her with options for healthier ways of living. But, even though by following the advice she did experience the benefits these changes brought to her life, she was so immersed in our disease-centric culture, so scared to address her real personal problems, she returned to her old habits rather than take responsibility for her life choices. As a result, she relinquished control over her own life to the system—with disastrous results.

TWO ALTERNATE ENDINGS

I began treating Melanie, a very bright and highly energetic forty-six-year-old mother of three, a few years ago. The first time she came to see me, she said she just wanted my opinion on her general regimen of care. Melanie told me she was suffering with a chronic case of Lyme disease, fibromyalgia, and possible multiple sclerosis. She was seeing experts for each one of the diseases in various cities around the country.

Through extensive and meticulous research, Melanie had found these experts, and in the process became so well-versed in this type of doctor research that she became the resource for referrals in health care for her community. Since she was around menopause and suffered with hot flashes, night sweats, insomnia and loss of libido she thought I would be a good doctor to help her integrate hormones with the overall care she was getting.

After spending a few hours talking to her and reading through the massive amount of records she brought to me, I asked her to connect me with the other healthcare practitioners involved in her life. She thought this was a strange question and explained that no other doctor had asked that before. When further prompted she told me that, in addition to the disease specialists, she was seeing an acupuncturist, a lymphatic massage therapist, a Reiki master, a naturopath, and a Chinese herbalist. When I asked about supplements, she produced a list of approximately fifty that she had been taking religiously at least twice a day for more than a decade.

I could not, in good conscience, prescribe another supplement or hormone for this poor woman. Her life was dominated by her conditions and the elaborate routines they required. I was concerned because interactions between different supplements may also cause health problems in spite of the benign status we perceive them to have. I strongly suggested she insist her doctors communicate with one another to coordinate her care. I also recommended she take a break from the supplements, herbs, and potions, and ask her doctors what would be the fallout of eliminating some of her medications. I suggested that after a few chemical, supplement, and doctor-free weeks, she reevaluate how she felt, at which point I'd be happy to help her figure out her next steps. Melanie was mortified by such an outlandish suggestion. She said she would think about it, but I never saw her again.

Fortunately, I can share a similar story with a more positive ending. Latisha is another patient of mine. She is also a mom in her early forties and, though not quite as extreme as Melanie, she too was taking large number of supplements and medications for a similar laundry list of conditions and syndromes. However, unlike Melanie, Latisha did choose to listen to me and encouraged her doctors to communicate. One called me crazy for recommending she take a holiday from the supplements, another filled her with fear about my "radical approach," but two of her doctors agreed to work with me. Latisha stopped the supplements, went off medications, and over the course of six months, the number of medical complaints she had dropped dramatically. As I began communicating with her doctors—she "fired" the ones who wouldn't speak to each other —and those left agreed to coordinate her care as a team. Five years later, she has just two physicians. She feels great and has told me, "Dr. E, I'm so happy with my life. I spend so much more time with my kids and friends, I never realized how much energy I was putting into being sick!" I hope that wherever she is, eventually, Melanie's story will lead to a similar happy ending.

TRAINING FOR DISEASE-CENTERED MEDICINE

The dehumanized and disease-centered healthcare system we have today continues to thrive largely because of the way physicians are trained. After four years of medical school and a few more years of postgraduate training and brainwashing, the newly minted doctor has sadly become a dehumanized version of his/her original self, without even realizing what happened. A once idealistic, caring young physician emerges from training without the understanding, guidance or experience to provide individualized care—even if s/he still wants to.

The word *brainwashing* in reference to medical education may seem like an exaggeration—perhaps the term 'coercive persuasion' would be easier to swallow—but the fact is there are more than a few frightening similarities between medical training and certain aspects of the indoctrination processes of cults and other groups that seek to reprogram the minds of their subjects. There have been extensive studies by sociologists and psychiatrists, beginning with the work of pioneers Robert J. Lifton and Edward Schein in the 1950s and 1960s with Korean War prisoners on this process. Enforced sleep deprivation, a reality for doctors in training since the profession began, is a core technique in brainwashing. Before physicians-in-training became unionized, via CIR (Committee of Interns and Residents), postgraduate training in county hospitals consisted of thirty-six-hour shifts on call, followed by twelve hours off. In large county hospitals, like Kings County where I trained, sleep was simply not an option for those on call. In fact, we used to talk about it; if you woke up in your own bed, you knew you wouldn't be sleeping for the next thirty-six hours. The least amount of work involved ward care, where you were on call every third night, but still had to care for more than fifty really sick patients that still meant no sleep.

Sleep deprivation is a universally known method of brainwashing and, yes, torture. It leaves an individual without the capacity to question authority or even think on his/her own. For the medical establishment, this produces an easily moldable intern and resident who accepts all information fed to him/her as fact. Another common brainwashing technique involves humiliation before one's peers, which has the multiple outcomes of intimidating the subject, destroying their self-confidence, and terrifying the rest of the group into full compliance. Attending physicians, who often have Godlike status in teaching hospitals, habitually berate interns and residents publically, leaving them too frightened to dare have a diverging opinion or to question the status quo. Another feature of coercive groups and cults is something called "milieu control," which is similar to what an abusive husband does when he gradually isolates his wife from her support system of friends and family. The mandatory eighty- to one hundred-hour work week required by medical education forces students to basically give up their nonmedical school-related activities and devote their lives pretty exclusively to their training. Friends, family, and hobbies are all moved to the back burner during medical school and postgraduate years. This kind of single-minded focus inevitably fails to produce well-rounded, compassionate doctors in favor of automatons who either forget basic social skills or never had the time to acquire them. Thus doctors emerge from medical school brainwashed and blindly following the authoritarian indoctrination they endured for four years. They are left with skewed perspectives on the doctor-patient relationship, blind trust in the educational process, and fear of questioning the status quo. Sadly this situation is the opening act that defines the rest of the doctor's interaction with the patients who unknowingly will entrust these newly minted doctors with their lives.

This idea of "medical training as a cult" is not something I made up. I once dropped in on and followed an online conversation between a group of doctors in training called SDN (Student Doctor Network).[16] A heated discussion was taking place among members questioning whether they felt they were being "brainwashed" by their medical education, and if they believed modern medicine might be similar to a cult. Some of those who posted scoffed angrily at the idea. Others had some very thoughtful and quite insightful observations.

One student put it most eloquently:

Medicine is more like a physically abusive relationship between a parent and child. The child hates the abuse growing up, but ends up being an abusive parent themselves. (Threepeas 03.30.06 – The Student Doctor Network)

THE EVOLUTION OF MEDICAL SCHOOL EDUCATION

In 1765, John Morgan at the University of Pennsylvania founded the first medical school in the original thirteen colonies known as the College of Philadelphia. It boasted a faculty trained at the University of Edinburgh and used British medical education as its model. Doctors in training learned hands-on, caring for the patients with their supervising physicians and sat in on classes and demonstrations in the operating theater. The medical school used the facilities at Pennsylvania Hospital, which was founded by Benjamin Franklin, and like most hospitals of the day, was a public health facility for the indigent and the acutely ill.

Medical education in that era included formal lectures for a semester or two and several years of clinical apprenticeship. There was no formal tuition, no prerequisite academic preparation, and written exams were not mandatory. Then in 1910, Abraham Flexner, a professional educator published the Flexner Report for the Carnegie Foundation. The report was a commentary on the state of medical education at the time. It criticized the fact that there were too many medical schools, many of which Flexner considered substandard. At the time, there were 155 medical schools in the United States and Canada and only sixteen of them required two or more years of college as prerequisite for admission. Flexner proposed a four-year medical school curriculum—two years of basic science, followed by two years of clinical training. Flexner's report forced many medical schools to close their doors because they did not have the means to adhere to Flexner's recommendations. Ironically, one hundred years after the Flexner Report, little has changed in the basic structure of medical school curriculum.

A LITTLE MORE ABOUT MEDICAL SCHOOL HISTORY

It should come as no surprise that the students of these early medical schools were mostly white and male. Totally segregated, there were only a few medical schools specifically for African-Americans. The first African-American to graduate from a northern medical school was Dr. David J. Peck, from Rush Medical School in 1847. Between 1868 and 1904, seven medical schools for African-Americans were established. Unfortunately, by 1923 only Howard University and Mehary Medical School remained open.

The situation wasn't much better for women. The first medical school for women, The Women's Medical College of Pennsylvania, was founded in 1850 and ultimately became co-ed and was renamed the Medical College of Pennsylvania. The first woman to graduate from a medical school in the U.S. was Dr. Elizabeth Blackwell, who graduated first in her class from Geneva Medical College in New York in 1849. The first African-American woman to graduate from a medical school in the U.S. was Dr. Rebecca Lee Crumpler who graduated from the New England Female Medical College in Boston in 1864.

While progress is being made, it is painfully slow. We are a heterogeneous society and we need our doctors to reflect the real face of our world if we are to provide truly excellent care to our patients.

THE MODERN MEDICAL SCHOOL

Today there are 150 accredited medical schools in the United States, all of which require MCATs (Medical College Admission Test) and a college degree as a prerequisite. Most medical schools still follow the curriculum proposed by Flexner more than one hundred years ago. When it comes to the gender and ethnic makeup of students, however, things have changed a bit. "Kaiser Health News (KHN) is a nonprofit news service committed to in-depth coverage of healthcare policy and politics. It reports on how the healthcare system – hospitals, doctors, nurses, insurers, governments, consumers – works." In 2011, KHN reported that about 7.7 percent of medical school graduates were Latino, 6.5 percent African American, 21.7 percent Asian, 0.8 percent Native American, and 62.1 percent Caucasian. The number of men and women graduating is finally about equal. The rest is still an uphill battle. No grades, GPA or MCAT score guarantee acceptance to a medical school and even graduating from a prestigious medical school doesn't guarantee you'll be a good doctor. It's a veritable minefield out there.

When I went to medical school in the 1970s at SUNY-Downstate College of Medicine (the only state school in New York City), there were thirty-five women in a class of 240 and there were only thirty-five African-Americans and three Asians in the class. The rest were white men—not that much different from the way it was in the 1920s. Other schools in New York at which I interviewed were even more rigid in their admissions of females or minority ethnic groups. In fact, I was interviewed at two very prestigious New York schools and although I had excellent grades and high MCAT scores, I was told point blank by my interviewers that they preferred male candidates since I was likely to get pregnant and drop out and would be wasting a precious medical school spot. In those days, there was no such thing as a discrimination suit. Senior doctors could say anything they wanted. They still do, only they couch their prejudice a little more carefully today.

STANDARDIZED HEALTH CARE

Standardized care is the general term descriptive of the use of protocols set by medical societies and specialty groups defining what is considered state-of-the-art practice of medicine. You've probably heard this term, either in your doctor's office, on the news, or TV medical dramas. Very simply, standardized care refers to conventionally sanctioned medical care in which the same treatment plans and practices are applied to patients with similar medical issues: treating elevated cholesterol levels with statins; checking PSA (prostate-specific antigen) levels yearly in men over fifty, or younger if they have a family history of prostate cancer, performing annual pap smears and mammograms; and when test results are abnormal, following the guidelines set by medical societies, follow up with biopsies, perform colonoscopies every 3-5 years after the age of fifty, annual physicals, etc.

This cookbook approach to medicine emerged as a necessity during the 19th century as part of medical school training as a way to create uniform care for indigent and acute or chronically ill patients. To this day it provides the basic ground rules for the practice of medicine. This is a good thing when used in the context of public health; but can be deadly if applied as a one-size-fits-all fix to all patients, ignoring the individual's specific needs and circumstance.

In the present climate, the standard of care implemented by doctors is likely to be influenced by pressures from drug companies, medical instrument companies, and insurance companies. Over the past few decades, the doctor's examination room has become very crowded. Every time you see the doctor, a collection of invisible forces influence his/her decisions and directly affect your care. Fear of malpractice suits and drug companies are all vying for a piece of the action and your doctor is either oblivious to or has accepted them as his masters in your care.

While medical training does teach young doctors to take a thorough history and examine the patient, by the time they get to the real practice of medicine, many have forgotten to look into the patient's eyes, to take the time to listen to the patient's personal story, and to ask about specific drugs, foods, or lifestyles that invariably affect the patient's medical status. The doctor has become a robot who follows protocols to serve special interest groups and protect him/herself from potential malpractice lawsuits. More and more the protocols of standardized care are set by corporations who don't care about the patient or his/her quality of life. In our thoroughly modern system, medical care is not about the patient—it's about the bottom line.

I don't believe there is a single doctor practicing today who hasn't been affected by the rigidity of medical care practiced under the aegis of standardized care and the disease-focused approach of modern medicine. I know I was, at first.

WHEN THE "RIGHT CALL" IS ALL WRONG

One night, while on night call during my second year of residency in internal medicine at Kings County Hospital in Brooklyn, I received a page from the Emergency Room to come down for an admission. The patient was an elderly woman in her seventies, who was in acute respiratory distress. My goal was to figure out what caused the distress and to treat her as swiftly as possible. I quickly realized the situation was dire and the woman was not going to make it. She had a pulmonary embolus—a large blood clot—in the main arteries to her lungs straddling the pulmonary arteries, something called a saddle embolus. It is a rare and deadly type of blood clot. Nothing I could have done would have saved her life. In that moment, I knew that the following morning I'd have to present her case at what was called "mortality and morbidity conference" to the head of the department and the entire staff consisting of students, junior and senior residents, and attending physicians. If I didn't have physical evidence of the cause of death, I would have had to wait for the autopsy report. I would have had to present my hypothesis for the cause of death of my patient because I had no proof of what really happened. That situation was a perfect set-up for humiliation and harsh criticism from the head of the department who was famous for his abusive treatment of the medical staff. The only way to avoid being embarrassed in front of my peers was to prove my diagnosis was correct. And the only way to do that was to get an angiogram while the patient was still alive. So at three o'clock in the morning I literally dragged the radiologist on call from his bed in the on-call room and begged him to perform an angiogram on the dying woman. She drew her last breath on the cold, hard angiography table. I had my proof in the form of the X-Ray, which showed the embolus sitting right at the point where the pulmonary arteries divide into left and right. My reputation saved, I proudly headed for the on-call room, after stopping by the waiting room to curtly tell the woman's husband that his wife of fifty years had passed away.

I was a good resident, conscientious and thorough. I had done my job with diligence and proved the diagnosis. My profession would be proud of me and during morning rounds I was a superstar. However, that incident became a tipping point in my life. The woman was my mother's age and her husband could have been my father. Did I want my parents to be treated the way I had treated this poor woman? I have relived that moment over and over again for decades. I suspected then, and I am certain now, that what I did was not the right thing, nor was it what modern standardized medical practice should be. My actions were insensitive and inhumane. The decent way to handle that situation would have been to sit down with the husband and tell him his wife was going to die; to tell him the truth about the reason why I wanted to have the angiogram; to allow husband and wife to be together for the few hours she had left in the privacy of a hospital bed in a quiet room. I didn't have to prove my diagnosis. Does it really matter what caused the final blow? I think what matters more is the kindness we choose to live our lives with.

DRUG COMPANIES MOVE IN

Medical care has taken two tracks. One is public health care focused on treating large populations and the other is individualized health focusing on treating one patient at a time. The shift from providing health care that focuses on the individual to a system that focuses on huge populations—public health—took a serious turn with the direction of medical training during the 1960s. Public health requires standardized protocols to help large numbers of people. To treat them drug companies saw the opportunity and started to develop standardized drugs in massive quantities. This led to the increasingly powerful position pharmaceutical companies achieved over the span of twenty-five years. In the process, pharmaceutical companies learned that mass-market blockbuster drugs generate hundreds of millions of dollars in revenue. This outcome quickly changed pharma from an altruistic industry looking to provide as many people as possible with life-saving drugs to a financially driven industry. Strangely, no federal regulation was ever instituted to curb the growing influence of dominion of big pharmaceutical companies over the practice of medicine. Money became the most important factor. This left physicians and hospitals financially dependent on their relationships with Big Pharma and most became victims of The Big Pharmaceutical takeover. The patient fell to the bottom of the priority list because money rules this system, not quality patient care.

WHERE'S THE BLACK BAG?

Modern medical training is about as far from caring about the individual patient as you can even imagine. It's like a nightmare. After four years of medical school and several more years of postgraduate training, the newly minted MDs no longer see their patients as individuals; their training insures the individual patient disappears in the haze of subspecialties, drugs, tests and procedures.

CHAPTER 3
WELCOME TO THE MEDICAL INDUSTRIAL COMPLEX

"Today's medicine is at the end of its road. It can no longer be transformed, modified, readjusted. That's been tried too often. Today's medicine must DIE in order to be reborn. We must prepare its complete renovation."

—Maurice Delort

If you've ever found yourself overwhelmed and confused as you navigate the fragmented, badly broken, and often-dangerous American healthcare system, you're not alone. The booming insurance industry, pharmaceutical corporations, and medical equipment companies, who together make up what is now known as the Medical Industrial Complex, have all conspired (and I'm not a conspiracy theorist) to create an environment that turns you—the patient—into its "perfect victim." It is a system about profit, first and foremost, rather than health, wellbeing, and your care.

Adding insult to injury, instead of representing your interests and acting as a frontline advocate in this mess, your doctor may very well have enlisted in the army of the enemy. Motivated by ego, trained to detach rather than to connect, terrified of malpractice suits, and following the guidance of medical societies motivated by fear of changing laws, insurance reimbursements, malpractice suits, fully bought by special interests and financially-driven conflicts of interest, too many doctors willingly become marionettes controlled by the puppet master the Medical Industrial Complex is. Maybe the doctors don't mean to become Medical Industrial Complex representatives, but unfortunately in our present world, most of them are just that. In following this dangerous path, they often inadvertently endanger their patients, who, struggling to make crucial decisions that will significantly and permanently impact their quality of life, are left at their mercy.

I believe many of my fellow physicians have lost sight of our primary purpose. No matter what public health or medical training would have you believe, the truth is that every human being is different, and every patient is first and foremost a unique human being with unique thoughts, feelings, problems and life situations. Physicians are bound by the Hippocratic Oath to begin every professional encounter with a patient by honestly asking ourselves, "What is the best I can do for the patient sitting in front of me?" If the doctor doesn't see you as a unique and separate individual from the statistics and public health training he/she has, chances are more likely that the physician will harm you than help you.

I don't want to believe that most doctors are more concerned with their bottom line than their patients' wellbeing. I know I'm an optimist, but I can't imagine any physician could ever put money ahead of the health of a patient. I believe most of us choose medicine as a profession, a life calling, because we genuinely want to help, not just to reap a financial windfall. Unfortunately, the problem is a lot more insidious than what we perceive as cynicism or greed. Physicians develop a belief system over decades of training and exposure to the practices of the traditional medical establishment, a desire to belong, and a pervasive refusal to question the status quo. Just like we aren't trained to see patients as individuals, doctors aren't trained to think independently. They are taught to follow "protocols," "evidence based medicine," and act robotically, almost thoughtlessly in "group think" fashion when treating human beings. Those who don't follow the party line established by medical societies are quickly ejected or marginalized from the system and become outsiders. They are considered *alternative*, unacceptable to the mainstream, and labeled quacks or snake oil salesmen with impunity and venom. Even if these outliers raise valid questions and challenge the wisdom of the status quo, the indoctrinated mainstream physician is conditioned to automatically reject the validity of an opposing point of view. Physicians for the most part are skeptics who don't listen—a deadly combination.

GETTING OFF THE MERRY GO ROUND

A forty-four year old patient of mine fell into the trap that awaits anyone who has blind faith in the system and reacts out of fear. Sadly, she hasn't made it out yet.

When I first met her, Lauren was a vivacious and charismatic international salesperson for a software company. She was also a newlywed, full of excitement for her new life with her new husband. She had a history of minor stomach issues, some hemorrhoids, and a low-functioning thyroid—a fairly common and non-life threatening medical issue which ran in her family. Otherwise, she was perfectly healthy.

Lauren traveled constantly for work and her husband was bicoastal for his career, so the two spent more time on a plane—both together and separately—than they did at home. About a year into married life, Lauren started complaining of fatigue. Her internist sent her for blood work and discovered she was anemic. Because her circulating iron, iron stores, and red blood cell parameters (the size and shape of which are affected by iron content) were normal on the blood test, it became clear her anemia wasn't caused by a simple iron deficiency.

To be safe, and following the guidelines of standardized care, the internist sent her to a hematologist. The hematologist performed further analysis of her blood cells and, finding the white blood cells to be marginally abnormal, ordered more detailed tests. When those also proved to be a little outside the standard reference range, he decided to do a bone marrow biopsy, which in turn showed more strange cells. The hematologist then recommended Lauren go to an academic center with a department specializing in the type of strange cells she had in her bone marrow. While at the center, she was referred to a rheumatologist, who was part of a twenty-doctor team dedicated to researching mysterious and stubborn autoimmune diseases, which Lauren guessed—but was never officially told—she had.

During her workup with the team, Lauren mentioned to one of the doctors that her periods weren't as regular or as light as they used to be. The team requested a gynecological consult. The gynecologist arrived promptly and ordered an ultrasound that showed a mass in her uterus. This prompted a uterine biopsy. The pathology report raised the possibility of a lymphoma—a cancer of blood cells located throughout the body's lymphatic system, usually specific to immune system cells. Next, as part of the lymphoma work-up and because of her history of a low-functioning thyroid, the team ordered a CT scan of the thyroid gland, which revealed lots of scarring. This was most likely due to the suppressed thyroid function, which had been successfully treated with thyroid hormones for decades. Just to be safe, the doctors ordered a thyroid biopsy. The biopsy was negative but as a side effect, the doctor injured a blood vessel in the thyroid gland and as result there was some bleeding at the site of the biopsy and Lauren developed a big swollen bruise on her neck. On another day Lauren mentioned to one of her many physicians that she had been having some problems with her vision—over the past three years her ophthalmologist had to gradually increase the strength of her contact lenses. Before she knew it, a team of ophthalmologists was on her case, evaluating her in depth and looking for a possible lymphoma in her right eye. The investigation continued and, as more doctors got involved, more problems were discovered. Some appeared to be serious, others less so, but all seemed to require further testing. The testing became more and more extensive and expensive. The innumerable visits to ever expanding numbers of specialists took over Lauren's entire life. This process continued for six months, while nothing was actively done to alleviate the original symptom—fatigue.

By this point, Lauren was even more tired than when she initially went to see her internist. The stress had deeply affected her sleep, her diet and she now suffered from severe fear and anxiety, and she had stopped exercising because she was depressed and sure she was going to die soon. In fact, she hardly had a waking moment that she wasn't worrying about her growing number of medical conditions. The stress caused her to lose twenty pounds and she began taking massive doses of sleeping pills and anxiety medications to get even a couple of hours of restless sleep. One of the doctors she told about the sleep issue sent her to a psychiatrist, who after spending fifty minutes with her placed her on an antidepressant. He told her he often saw people in situations like hers, who were depressed and needed medication—even if only for a short period of time.

I originally started seeing Lauren to help her with the low thyroid, and also focus her on healthy nutrition and exercise balance so she could feel and look her best for her then upcoming wedding. When she next came to see me, she looked terrible, and I learned of the relentless medical gauntlet she was running. Wanting to do anything to help, I asked her to allow me to compare notes with her coordinating doctor at the academic center. Lauren thought that was a great idea, but couldn't tell me who that person was. She truly had no idea. There were so many doctors, nurses, assistants, and technicians involved in her case that she had lost track. Lauren was understandably scared and confused. The last I heard from her, she still had no clear diagnosis—despite ongoing visits and expert care from one of the most respected academic centers in the country for more than six months.

It seemed obscene to me that this strong, intelligent woman had entrusted her care to the top doctors in the country in the hopes of finding the cause of her fatigue, yet not one of these doctors treated her as whole human being. There was no doctor in charge helping her put all the pieces together, no one coordinating an integrated treatment plan to help her regain her life. She was more exhausted than ever, having to make up work time lost to medical appointments with more red-eye flights and weekend sessions.

Since I've only seen a handful of isolated test results—sporadically sent to me by some of her doctors—I can't say for sure what is wrong with Lauren. Of course, it is possible that all these horrific medical problems had simultaneously besieged this one unlucky young woman. Or, it could be that she was simply unlucky enough to become tangled up in a complex web of tests and biopsies at the wrong time in her life? Maybe we all have significant problems that exist in our bodies at certain times, but left alone maybe over time our bodies heal without medical intervention, allowing us to go on with our lives? Perhaps if we looked at the problems Lauren experienced while under the care of the academic center from a slightly different perspective, an entirely different picture might emerge. Lauren's worsening eyesight is a common sign of aging that seems to accelerate when we are stressed or tired. A decrease in visual acuity often begins in the late-thirties to mid-forties, but eventually evens out in most people. Lauren was forty-four, so she was right on track for this normal aging problem. Peri-menopause can start for some women as early as the mid-thirties, most commonly in women like Lauren, who live type-A, stress-filled lives. By forty-four, many women are well on their way to losing their sex hormones and entering menopause, which would account for the change in her menstrual cycle. During this period in a woman's life cycle, hormones start changing and the symptoms that ensue are often confused with disease, when in fact they are just the body responding to natural hormonal fluctuations. So what could be the cause of her original complain of fatigue? In addition to the hormone changes and the low thyroid she'd had for decades, it could also be that all those late nights of arduous work, the constant travel, never-ending time zone changes, dietary shifts, and lack of exercise were wreaking havoc not just on her sleep cycles. Perhaps some lifestyle changes would have been a safer and gentler first order of treatment, before she was shuffled onto the medical testing merry-go-round. Perhaps, if she and her first doctor had originally discussed her slightly abnormal blood tests as two people in a partnership committed to making Lauren's quality of life the highest priority, they might have decided on a less aggressive strategy. Perhaps they would have opted to make lifestyle changes first, waiting to repeat the tests again in a few weeks or months, instead of immediately running to specialists, biopsies and dramatic and scary diagnosis. Perhaps if they had done all that, Lauren's outcome would have been totally different.

But then, fear-based medical care requires immediate action for every potential problem. *Get to the bottom of it! Do all the tests! Medicate it! Take it out!* It takes a strong patient—and a courageous doctor—to swim against the current, to focus on the big picture, to make decisions using common sense and not fear.

Too many people, once convinced there is something wrong with them, will refuse to let go of the notion of illness and let the body take care of itself. There will always be a doctor, a system, an academic center willing and able to perpetuate the fear and determined to find something wrong that needs treatment.

Another huge problem is the insurance status. Most people look upon good insurance coverage as essential, but for Lauren, and too many like her, it has the potential to become a highly negative influence on their medical care. Lauren had excellent, comprehensive insurance through her high-powered position at work. Once an insurance company is willing to pay for a system run amok, you are at risk of being broken down into millions of tiny little pieces, each with individual labels, without a clear treatment plan and absolutely no perspective or interest in improving your quality of life. It's like donating your body to science while you're still alive.

THE RISE OF THE INSURANCE MONOPOLY

While we all complain and see the horrors of our insurance system, it's important to understand that insurance companies existed in health care for many decades and they once worked for the benefit of the patient. Before the rise of the insurance-monopoly in the healthcare system, in the 1980's, there were commercial insurances some people who had the means or job position could afford. There were also government-sponsored insurance programs, like Medicare for the elderly and Medicaid for the underprivileged. Beyond that, most patients paid reasonable fees for doctor's visits and testing. The prices weren't nearly as high as they are now.

I remember when I opened my first internal medicine private practice in the mid-1980s, in a suburb of New York City, the annual physical exam—which was recommended and religiously implemented then, but is in question now[17]—cost $150 and regular office visits ranged from $25-$30. Patients paid with cash or check and there was no incentive to order extravagant treatments or testing, nor was there fear of malpractice.

I remember one middle-aged patient—I'll call him Charlie—who always came to my practice in his red Porsche, which he parked in front of my office. Comprehensive and capitated (a fixed, predetermined monthly payment received by a physician, clinic, or hospital per patient) insurance coverage were just coming into existence and I wasn't sure whether to join the trend. Some of our patients, who were teachers, had asked us to accept GHI (the insurance provided by their union), so our office manager enrolled us.

One day, after a routine visit, Charlie and I walked to the checkout area of my office. As I watched him hand a five-dollar bill to our secretary, I asked him why he was only paying $5 for the visit. He told me that his wife had GHI insurance, which we were now accepting, and he was on her policy. I'm a very direct person, so I told him I felt being paid $5 for my services didn't feel right, since it was devaluing my work as his doctor. He said, "But you accept the insurance." He also told me he didn't intend to offend me and would pay whatever it took to keep me as his doctor. I will forever be grateful to Charlie in the red Porsche. He opened my eyes to what was to come and I was lucky to have the self-confidence to refuse to take insurance ever again. You have no idea how easy it is for any doctor, under the threat of losing patients and the competitive whining of peers, to drown in the impersonal insurance shuffle and wind up serving the insurance master rather than the patient. I told my office manager to get out of GHI and never joined another insurance plan. I strongly and undoubtedly believe the relationship between the patient and doctor should not be influenced by insurance, drug and equipment companies, or fear of malpractice. Anyone that comes between the doctor and the patient is going to deter from optimal patient care.

Even in today's age of specialized medicine, success is still primarily linked to relationships and consistency of care. Study after study[18] has shown that the best health care—from patients on Medicaid, to pay-as-you-go patients, to those who participated in the early experimental HMOs (like "Romneycare" in Massachusetts during the early 1980s)—always comes down to one thing and one thing only: coordinated care that is based on a solid, consistent relationship between patient and primary care physician. That is the BEST care.

We should have learned that lesson from practical experience back in the era of the commonsense house call. However, once HMO-mania caught on, that lesson went out the window. Insurance companies smelled money—big money—so care was reduced to assembly lines and numbers. And what happened then? According to John Abramson MD, author of *Overdosed America: The Broken Promise of American Medicine*[19], healthcare costs per person (adjusted for inflation) have more than quadrupled in twenty years. Starting in 2001, premiums rose 43 percent over the following three years alone. And, along with rising costs, came radically deteriorating outcomes. America started falling further and further behind other industrialized countries in crucial areas of medical care, such as infant mortality and life expectancy—the U.S. ranks 26th right behind Slovenia.[20] The United States has a higher infant mortality rate than any of the other twenty-seven wealthy countries according to a new report from the Centers for Disease Control. A baby born in the US is nearly three times as likely to die during her first year of life as one born in Finland or Japan. That same American baby is about twice as likely to die in her first year as a Spanish or Korean baby.[21] At the same time, we suffer among the highest rates of heart disease, Type 2 diabetes, and obesity. A 2014 study in the journal *The Lancet* confirmed again that the US is the most overweight country on Earth. Compared to 38 percent of men and 36.9 percent of women worldwide who are overweight or obese, 70.9 percent of men and 61.9 percent of women fall into that category in the United States[22]. We also have the seventh highest cancer rate in the world.[23] As for the U.S. famed *War on Cancer*—including all our "astounding medical breakthroughs," our innumerable "Walks for the Cure," and our gleaming multibillion dollar cancer centers—only serve to perpetuate a myth of medical superiority that is plain unfounded.

Pandora's box has been opened. Almost out of the gate, insurance and pharmaceutical companies diverted a large chunk of their astronomical profits to advertising budgets, ensuring no one ever questions the status quo. News of more medical "breakthroughs" and the promise of perfect health in a pill—in genomics and proteomics—are marketed to the American public on a daily basis and we happily buy into this myth hook, line, and sinker and, all too often, end up paying with our lives.

FOOLS IN THE GAME

When it comes to the manipulative way insurance companies have wormed their way into and ultimately monopolized modern medicine, doctors are the smallest part of the conspiracy. Under the current system, doctors work for the insurance companies (as well as the drug companies and medical equipment companies you'll read about in the next chapters). Once you find a doctor you like, you're going to have to get on an insurance plan that he or she takes. When the insurance monopoly began, doctors got on board out of fear—fear of losing patients, fear of being ostracized, fear of being outsiders when everyone else was joining in. And you can be sure all these fears were deliberately instilled in doctors by the insurance companies, their medical society peers, and the legal ramifications of not following "standard of care" (just as the fear of being sick or missing the diagnosis of a potentially deadly disease is instilled in patients). Like most of us, doctors are subject to the herd mentality, and thus, unable to foresee the behemoth the insurance industry would eventually become, blindly accepted the new rules of a game no one understood.

Today, just like the consumer, doctors have become victims of corporate greed. When insurance companies started chipping away at doctor's reimbursements, limiting payments, rejecting claims, and devaluing their work, doctors began to strike back. Little by little, they figured out how to play the system to their advantage. What's come out of this is a game—the game of documentation— that has spiraled out of control while it is keeping thousands employed and further eroding the quality of health. This is how it works: based on the standard diagnostic guidelines in every medical specialty, every known illness, condition, syndrome, diagnosis and therapy, surgical procedure, radiologic procedure, etc. has been given a number and classification. These are known as ICD (International Classification of Diseases), CPT (Current Procedural Terminology), and DMS (Diagnostic Statistical Manual of Mental Disorders) codes. When a doctor examines a patient, s/he records the information and diagnosis in the patient's chart. A coder, typically a secretary or billing expert, then assigns the appropriate diagnostic and procedure the codes, preferably ones that command the highest reimbursement rate. Insurance companies base their decision to approve or deny treatment entirely on those codes. It doesn't take much reflection to see the fatal flaw in this system: once a visit to the doctor or a course of treatment becomes a recorded code, the patient no longer matters—s/he becomes nothing more than a set of numbers and classifications. An entire industry of expert consultants, who give courses on expert coding to doctors offices, clinics, and hospitals, has emerged to help get the most money out of the insurance company. As long as the record is expertly coded and the documentation supports the code, insurance companies will pay. Quality of patient care is truly irrelevant.

Doctors, who clearly benefit from this terribly dishonest and inefficient method of providing medical care, never question the system, so long as they are not penalized for overdoing the coding. A slap on the wrist or small fine closes the book on much of the fraud that permeates the system. There are no safeguards or incentives to be honest and provide good patient care. Only documentation and coding matter. A sad state of affairs.

TRADING LIVES FOR REIMBURSMENTS

Sadly too many doctors tempted by easy money, choose the wrong path to follow. All you have to do is read the newspaper. Rarely does a week go by that a doctor doesn't get caught fraudulently extracting monies from insurance companies by taking advantage of the coding and documentation loopholes. Most do it in underprivileged areas, where assembly-line medicine prevails. But there are others, even in top academic institutions, who abuse the system in plain sight.

I practice medicine in New York City, a Mecca for advanced medical care. Somewhere in my city, there is a group of ob-gyns that brings in a lot of money to the University Hospital they refer their patients to. The practice is made up of young female doctors, and the group is primarily motivated by financial incentives not care or compassion for its patients. The doctors routinely frighten pregnant women into unnecessary procedures often times because the insurance companies pay higher reimbursement rates when the doctor classifies a patient as high risk. This is just one of the many horrific side effects of the documentation game and the lack of ethics in the profession. But the story doesn't end with pregnant women. In this elite group, all women are potential prey to these dishonorable doctors.

One of the group's former patients told me the following story:

Arlette was in her twenties when she had her first abnormal pap smear. She had been infected with HPV (a common, sexually transmitted virus that is usually self-limited and is similar to the common cold. It has numerous strains of which more than 90% resolve on their own. A small percentage stays in the system and is associated with a higher risk of cervical cancer if not properly watched with regular gyn follow-ups). Her particular strain was one of the few that doesn't resolve spontaneously and if left unattended for decades, carries an increased risk of cervical cancer. Arlette was a very conscientious patient, who followed up with Pap smears every six months. Most were negative, but once in a while she had a mildly abnormal result, for which she was treated with a colposcopy (a procedure that closely examines the cervix, vagina, and vulva for signs of disease) followed by LEEP (Electrosurgical Excision Procedure) to remove any abnormal cervical tissue. By the time she was thirty-eight, her Pap smear tests had been consistently normal for more than five years. In the sixth year, after a mildly abnormal Pap result, the senior physician in the group told her it was time for a hysterectomy. When Arlette asked why she couldn't continue the routine she had been following for decades, her doctor flippantly told her she was getting old, most likely wasn't going to have children and insisted it was a perfect time for the hysterectomy. Also, Arlette had great insurance with her current employer, which would cover the expense of the procedure, so her doctor thought this was a great opportunity that she may not have with the next job. Mortified by the cavalier attitude of the doctor, a woman doctor who she felt should have been more sympathetic, Arlette ran out of the office, never to return again. She began seeing another gynecologist, a man, who performed her LEEP and now, six years later, at forty-five, she still has her uterus and normal Paps. In fact, two years ago, she had a baby with the help of a fertility doctor who supported her throughout the entire process.

Here are two other stories from former patients of the same ob-gyn group:

Hailey was a pregnant woman whose ob-gyn, in the same practice, told her she could have diabetes because she had gained too much weight, according to statistics without ever asking about her family history. Even though her blood tests for diabetes were all normal, nor did she have any symptoms of diabetes (thirst, frequent urination, dry mouth), the doctor insisted she undergo extensive and uncomfortable testing to rule out diabetes. (Keep in mind: insurance companies pay higher fees for what is labeled as "high risk pregnancy.") Diabetes, or the risk of diabetes creates a "high risk pregnancy" leading to a change in the diagnosis code and insurance pays a higher reimbursement than a normal pregnancy. Hailey had a brother who was a doctor and he recommended she leave the group and find a kinder, more caring doctor. She left the practice in the thirty-fifth week of her normal pregnancy. She never heard from the doctor although she did receive an insurance report on a claim submitted by the practice long after she no longer used the doctor.

Geneva and her husband had been unsuccessfully trying to get pregnant for six months. She told the doctor she saw in the group that she was considering seeing a fertility specialist. The doctor recommended Geneva have an ultrasound performed in the doctor's office. Soon after, the doctor returned to the examining room and confidently told Geneva she had a small fibroid in her uterus that was very likely the reason she wasn't getting pregnant. She said matter-of-factly that she would remove it with a minor surgical procedure, which would make it easy for Geneva to get pregnant without expert help. Geneva was suspicious and decided to go for a second opinion. She went to see a fertility expert, who told her that the fibroid was tiny and had nothing to do with her difficulty getting pregnant. He also told Geneva not to worry because all the tests had come back normal and she should go on vacation with her husband. The couple went to the Florida Keys and got pregnant—fibroid and all—shortly thereafter. The insistence on the removal of the fibroid was yet another insurance scam; more surgical procedures also translate into higher reimbursement rates for the doctors and hospital.

Finally, after some further in depth investigation by my office due to the multiple complaints about this particular ob-gyn practice we received, it turned out that the practice had the highest rate of Caesarian sections in New York City. The chairman of their department at the academic institution they practice out of is quite aware of the shady practices of this group—and the many complaints filed by patients and their families—but he chooses to ignore them because the group is a top "producer" and fills hospital beds and operating rooms. A tough choice: reprimand bad care or turn a blind eye to fraudulent practices that generate revenue for the hospital.

THE CHOICE

Not all doctors follow this dark path of dishonesty and negligent care. There are doctors who put together like-minded doctor groups, decide to stop taking insurance, and place the wellbeing of the patient ahead of the money or the intimidation of special interest groups. The decision where you stand as a doctor is a choice made by every responsible medical professional at some point in his or her career. Who are you here to serve: the Medical Industrial Complex or the patient? One way or another, each one of us in the medical profession has to look in the mirror and make that choice.

Personally, I faced that choice in my mid-thirties. After five years of running the emergency room of an academic trauma center, I opened my own private practice. I started out as a conventional internist. I had been trained and indoctrinated well. I believed everything I had been taught. But within a couple of years in practice, I noticed that all I was doing was ordering tests and performing physical exams. I sent most of my patients home just as they came, with no help to improve their lives. I would tell them to come back in three or six months to repeat tests, hoping that eventually I would find something seriously wrong and come up with a disease to justify performing more tests and prescribing more medications, many of which were samples from pharmaceutical reps who relentlessly inundated my office. Coming out of a specialty in emergency medicine, it felt disingenuous to wait for healthy people to get sick. I wanted to help, but the way I was practicing medicine was doing nothing to prevent disease. All I did was waste time and money waiting for disease to manifest itself in my patients. So after a couple of years of struggling to do what I had been taught, I began to change.

First, I shed my white coat. I felt it did less to keep me from getting blood or other body secretions on my clothes, than it did to create distance between my patients and me. It made me appear different from them, the mighty doctor, not their partner in their health care as I wanted to be. Next, I began asking more questions about their lives. I asked about their personal lives, work, and family. Little by little, I began to make surprising connections between stress and disease. It became clear to me that if I knew my patients and their life stressors, I could anticipate times when they were at risk of getting sick and could offer them commonsense tools to prevent or shorten the duration of illnesses as simple as colds and flu. I took graduate courses in nutrition and fitness and began giving advice in areas no conventional doctor usually bothers with, areas that directly impact everyday life.

More than a few of my colleagues from the academic centers where I had worked before opening my practice thought I was losing my mind. Some questioned if I was becoming a psychiatrist, others gossiped that I was crossing over to a career in alternative medicine—something sadly disdained by traditional MDs.

I reassured them that I was simply doing what every good conventional doctor needs to do: expand his/her horizons and focus on figuring out how to help their patients improve their lives.

One day, a patient with a terrible backache came to see me. In those days, the conventional "standard of care" protocol for backaches was to prescribe a muscle relaxant, an anti-inflammatory, and a few days of bed rest. Instead—just acting out of instinct and the new perspective I had on my role as a doctor—I got down on the floor with the patient and showed her some gentle stretches I had learned from the trainers I worked with and a physical therapist patient. Even though I told her my recommendation was totally unorthodox, she wanted to try it. The result was nothing short of amazing. She stood up slowly and, mouth agape, told me she felt much better. That was the first time I dared to deviate from conventional medical practice and the result gave me courage and incentivized me to continue on my new path.

I helped another patient consider serious dietary changes because he was overweight and, according to his blood results, "pre-diabetic." He had tried numerous diets, but couldn't stick with them and they didn't really help lower his blood sugar levels. Together, we worked on creating a diet to fit into his lifestyle that he could stick with. His blood sugar levels dropped to normal as he quickly lost ten pounds. Another patient with high blood pressure and marital strife took my recommendation to lower the stress in her marriage by going into counseling with her husband. Again, the medical problem (high blood pressure) resolved without medication. The more connections I made between lifestyle, diet, exercise, and stress, the better I was able to help my patients with commonsense advice and the results were nothing short of miraculous across the board.

As I learned how to listen better, to understand my patients as people, as unique humans and most importantly to leave my ego out of the examining room, I gradually left the disease-centered model of health care in my rear view mirror. A limitless horizon of patient-centric, prevention-focused practice lay before me.

THE DISAPPOINTMENT OF OBAMACARE

The Affordable Care Act—otherwise known as Obamacare—was supposed to help every American get insurance and better health care. In the summer of 2009 when Obamacare made its grand entrance in our healthcare system, I was consulting for a small insurance company, focused on prevention. As part of my job, I participated in media round-table discussions on health care. The participants, mostly physicians with administrative positions and insurance representatives, were all trying to understand and explain to the public how the Affordable Care Act was going to help reign in out of control expenses and help provide insurance to millions of uninsured Americans. I started out genuinely believing that Obamacare was going to be a powerful and much needed solution. I thought that if the issue of insurance was taken off the table—if everyone had insurance—then the focus of health care would shift back to the patient, to better quality of care. I naïvely assumed Obamacare would help move health care toward the desperately needed patient-centric, prevention-based model.

Regrettably, I was wrong. By the second week of the healthcare conversation, President Obama—whom I'd voted for precisely because he professed to care about the American public—started meeting behind closed doors with the policy makers who would shape the ACA: first in line were the insurance companies and a close second were representatives of the drug companies. To my enormous disappointment, once again, doctors and patients were at the bottom of the list. So much for the revolution in medicine that Obamacare had promised. The best thing that can be said about Obamacare is that it has allowed some people who were denied insurance because of preexisting conditions to get some sort of coverage. But, overall, it has further increased the power of insurance companies, created more confusion, and lowered quality of care even more. A patient-centric system that focuses on the patient and prevention of disease is still a dream.

THE MYTH OF "GREAT INSURANCE"

The politics of health insurance have led a majority of people to believe that good insurance coverage equals good health care. I've often heard patients say, "Doctor, please order anything you want, I have great insurance and they will pay for anything. I'd like a few more tests, *just in case.*"

This is such a dangerous way of thinking. People believe that the insurance company is helping them get access to better medical care, but nothing could be further from the truth. It's each and every one of us who pay for every single benefit covered by insurance. From the CEO of the insurance company, who makes hundreds of millions of dollars (mostly in bonuses), to the claims adjustors and clerks paid to reject as many claims as possible, each and every one of us pays their salaries and at the same time we are their victims as they perpetuate this overwhelming deception every day.

If people understood that we pay to make insurance companies rich and they don't pay to keep us healthy, they might rise up against the system and dismantle it for good. I won't mince words, I believe the corporate-owned insurance system has created a dangerous situation and has contributed to the deplorable health care we have now. Total federal spending on health care eats up nearly 18 percent of the nation's output, about double what most other industrialized nations spend on health care. The last thing corporate insurance does is provide protection or care for the patient. The young pay to cover the old, the costs of whose care in the last six months of life are astronomical and actually make up the highest percentage of healthcare costs in the nation. In 2011, Medicare spending reached close to $554 billion, which amounted to 21 percent of the total dollars spent on U.S. healthcare in that year. Of that $554 billion, Medicare spent 28 percent or about $170 billion, on patients' last six months of life.[24] I am totally in favor of providing health care and serious, caring support to every aging American. I'm not advocating the elimination of Medicare or any other federally subsidized healthcare system. I am trying to bring to light the misrepresentation and misuse of funds that is endemic in our healthcare system. In my extensive experience, the current system abuses and takes advantage of the old. More surgeries, procedures, and drugs are performed on people in the last year of life than is ethical, honest or caring. When we know a person is terminally ill, there is no moral reason to use them to milk the system for more money by doing more to them. The biggest fraud in the system is when families of dying patients are told that one more test, one more procedure may extend the lives of a loved one by another day or another month. Subjecting a dying patient to more invasive tests and procedures robs them of quality of life in their final days. This abuse affects entire families and denies the patient a kind and gentle acceptance of the fact that we are all mortal and cannot avoid death.

The issue of exploitation in end-of-life care is worthy of its own book. Senior citizens, our parents and grandparents (and, sooner or later, each one of us), deserve far better than to be relegated to an impersonal hospital ward at the end of a long life filled with hard work and beautiful contributions to our children and to our country. The unbridled greed of insurance companies, hospitals, and Big Pharma makes a mockery of the Old Testament commandment to "honor thy father and thy mother." Whether you're an atheist, Christian, Jew, Muslim, Hindu, Buddhist, Wiccan, or secular humanist, this moral imperative is more than religious doctrine, it is a basic tenant of human decency that crosses cultural and geographic borders. But, as Vicki's sister's story from Chapter 1 illustrates, it's being violated every day by the heartless Medical Industrial Complex. It's an outrage, it's inhumane, and we're all contributing to it with our policy dollars and our passive fearful stance toward insurance and health care in general.

As far as insurance goes, there are really only three types the average, healthy person can use:

1) Catastrophic insurance: This covers you if you are in an accident, have a heart attack or stroke, or need any kind of acute care. The cost of this insurance is low for young people. It increases with age, but is generally affordable throughout life. The deductible is known up front so you can set aside that amount, put it in the bank, and ideally, not have to touch it unless you really need it.

2) Health savings account (HSA): A tax-deductible medical savings account available to taxpayers in the United States who are enrolled in a high-deductible health plan (HDHP) or choose not to have insurance. The funds contributed to this type of account are not subject to federal income tax at the time of deposit. Sometimes your employer may choose to participate and pay a portion of it. With this option, you put in the same amount you would pay for insurance premiums, except that the money is held in a bank in escrow instead of going to the insurance company. You use it as an expense account when you need medical care. People who make this out-of-the-box choice consistently find they have money in the bank at the end of the year.

3) Long-term care insurance: This type of coverage becomes necessary when, either as the result of a catastrophic incident or as you enter the end-of-life zone, you require extended nursing care to assist with basic daily activities, such as bathing, walking, or transferring from bed to chair. You can pay a much lower fee on a yearly premium that can be paid on a monthly basis if you get this insurance in your thirties and forties and when you need it decades later you have decent affordable coverage for long-term care, either in your home or in an assisted living facility. Long-term care gets activated when you have difficulty with activities of daily living.

The rest of insurance is nothing short of a brilliant scam, set up by the industry and integrated into our culture to justify a most profitable business and scare us into the need for coverage. Many of your visits to doctors and specialists, access to testing and other medical needs are covered inconsistently at best. In my experience I have seen patients with no insurance getting the best of care and patients with excellent insurance getting deprived of basic healthcare needs.

It is absolutely imperative that you read the fine print and take time to carefully review every policy you consider, because insurance companies are betting that you'll just sign on the dotted line and never understand your benefits under your policy. Hidden caveats that preclude you from getting the promised coverage even after you have been paying in for decades are the rule rather than the exception.

When it comes to choosing an insurance policy, if it seems too good to be true, you can pretty much bet it is. The following is a cautionary tale, told by my patient, Victoria Reggio, of another tragic example from her own life:

WHERE'S THE INSURANCE BENEFIT?

When my sister, Emily was in her forties, an insurance broker sold her a long-term health insurance policy. The policy would cover her needs should she become disabled and in need of in home or nursing home help. Emily signed up at her company's HR department's recommendation. She was told in no uncertain terms that it would be less expensive to do so at a younger age, rather than wait until her late fifties or sixties when it becomes prohibitive.

Emily was single, didn't have children, and was afraid of being unable to care for herself in her old age. These factors qualified her for this type of policy. For almost twenty years, Emily paid her premiums on a monthly basis and sure enough at the age of sixty-two, when she was hospitalized with terminal cancer, she needed this policy to provide her the financial support it promised. We contacted the insurance company to ask them to pay for the home health aids and services to assist her when she was released from the hospital. Remember, these were the key selling points that persuaded Emily to buy this insurance in the first place. Emily was a patient at the most prominent cancer hospital in the country and we provided documentation from the doctors and social workers that confirmed her need for long-term care to the insurance company. We assumed her case would be handled quickly and efficiently.

Not so. It took three months of faxing and repeated phone calls to the insurance company leading nowhere fast, before the policy was approved three days after my sister Emily passed away.

My sister had paid more than $100,000 dollars in premiums over twenty years yet she never saw a single dollar from them when she needed the policy to help her.

The very existence of the insurance industry and its draconian rules encourages both overuse and abuse, something both doctors and patients enable to and, though their motivations may be innocent, the results most often only benefit the insurance company.

Think about it: if you didn't have insurance, would you be so quick to get tests you may not need? And how would that impact your search for disease? Maybe asking the doctor who sends you for the test would be a good place to start. Missing a lump that turns out—like most— to be benign, diagnosing an unpreventable, chronic illness long before you experience symptoms—does that really delay treatment? Doesn't most medical care feel like a game of hurry-up-and-wait? Where is prevention in this system? What exactly are your doctors doing to help you prevent chronic diseases before they take hold? How often does your doctor explain in detail what "lose some weight" or "eat a healthier diet" means? How often does your doctor give you truly useful tips on how to exercise more efficiently? How often does your doctor talk to you about stress management or discuss the recent scientific studies revealing the crucial role of sleep in health maintenance? No test or medication will help you figure out a better way to live and even prevent illness.

THE HEARTBREAK OF HEARTBURN

Let's look at what might be a typical case, a compilation patient we'll call Joe. Joe is a forty-five-year-old man, who confides in a friend that lately he has been experiencing a lot of heartburn. Joe's friend immediately launches into a horror story he heard about someone's friend—or maybe it was something he read online. Whoever it was, the guy had heartburn that turned out to be stomach cancer and by the time it was discovered it had spread, killing the victim at fifty-two in literally three months, widowing his young wife and leaving his two small children fatherless.

That story would send most people with similar symptoms running to the doctor to make sure they weren't heading in the same situation. It's just human nature. I have seen dozens of people with similar stories in the ER and in my private offices. So Joe goes to his internist and tells him about the heartburn and adds, "Doctor, I'm really afraid there's something much more serious going on here."

Joe's dramatic pronouncement will likely make his internist very, very nervous. Not over any realistic fear that Joe might have a potentially deadly disease, because like most doctors, he has seen enough patients to feel pretty confident that Joe is a reasonably healthy guy and the percentage of patients whose heartburn is a serious symptom of some significant illness is extremely low. No, Joe's doctor is now afraid of Joe. He knows that if he doesn't protect himself, should he leave any stone unturned, something should turn out to be wrong with Joe, he is left wide open for a malpractice lawsuit for negligence and missed diagnosis. So, as "standard of care" dictates, Joe's doctor refers him to a gastroenterologist. Thus he dilutes his own risk exposure by pawning Joe off onto a specialist. The situation also enables another doctor to benefit financially from Joe's fear, and so the system thrives.

Joe arrives at the gastroenterologist's office and presents his insurance card to the receptionist. She smiles. Joe has great insurance and the doctor is in the plan! The gastroenterologist comes into the examination room and asks Joe to tell her his story, as it relates to the heartburn. She asks only questions that relate to the heartburn—she's a gastroenterologist so his esophagus, stomach, intestines, liver and pancreas are the only parts of Joe that concern her. How long has he had the heartburn? Does he smoke? Does he drink? What has he been taking for the heartburn? Has he seen any other doctors for the problem? Joe tells her his story and she promptly decides—based on his answers—that the next step for Joe is an upper endoscopy (also known as gastroscopy, this procedure involves placing a tube with a camera at its end into the stomach to evaluate the lining of the esophagus and stomach and to take samples—biopsies—of the stomach, esophagus and culture the contents for bacteria—where and when necessary). The procedure is performed by gastroenterologists routinely. She tells him that this is the best way to get to the heart of the matter. It will help figure out what could be causing his heartburn— a possible ulcer, an infection in the stomach, or worst-case scenario, some precancerous condition or even cancer.

Once Joe hears the word "cancer," the rest of the conversation goes on mute. The doctor's mouth is moving, but no sounds are coming out. It's like a scene in a horror movie when the soundtrack suddenly fades to white noise and everything starts happening in slow motion. Now, Joe is trembling with fear. Once the "C" word is on the table, all bets are off and he'll say "yes" to any test, any drug, any procedure.

Within a few weeks, Joe had the upper endoscopy, gastric motility studies (evaluation of how his stomach empties), and stomach and esophageal biopsies. The doctor keeps repeating that, "It's better to be safe than sorry."

But are all these tests really in Joe's best interest? No one asks that question, not Joe nor the gastroenterologist.

The strange yet very common problem is that no one has asked Joe some very basic questions. What's his diet like? Does he eat late at night? What about caffeine? Alcohol? What about recent stressors in his life or work? The gastroenterologist didn't even consider having Joe try a week or two on a less acidic, more alkaline (ph>7.5) diet (FYI, there is no nutrition course in any medical school curriculum and conventional doctors are specifically taught to be totally skeptical about the connection between nutrition and disease. Sadly, I'm not kidding). What about suggesting Joe try some over-the-counter antacids not to mention H2 inhibitors such as Zantac, Tagamet, or Pepcid? Come to think of it, why didn't Joe's primary care physician offer these simple and low-cost suggestions to see if things got better before resorting to specialist referrals, invasive testing, and biopsies? Before scaring Joe by raising the possibility of cancer, before using intimidation and panic to decide how best to provide medical care.

Let's also not forget about the role insurance plays in this all-too common yet pathologic scenario. Because Joe has such good insurance the specialist is more likely to recommend a plethora of testing. As a gastroenterologist, she makes her living off tests the like of gastroscopy (upper endoscopy) and biopsies. Insurance will only pay a couple of hundred dollars for a routine consultation, but when a couple of "safe" "recommended" "standard of care" procedures are added, the doctor will make thousands of dollars in short order. Doctors may be perceived as the pawns in the insurance game, but they too have learned how to squeeze out their share of the system. And they are doing it under the watchful eye of their professional societies that recommend and endorse aggressive testing as state-of-the-art medical practice.

As for the patient in this case, Joe, well, he still can't get that cancer story his friend told him out of his head. He lies in bed at night, his brain endlessly churning over the word—cancer, cancer, cancer. And to him, just like for millions of other people indoctrinated by our society, cancer means death. It means he won't be there for his kids' college graduations, their weddings, or live to enjoy retirement. Already, in his vivid imagination, his life is over. Plus, now Joe has had time to Google every possible worst-case scenario that could even remotely be connected to heartburn. He knows his insurance will pay and he wants every test in the book to make sure nothing is missed. Joe's gastroenterologist doesn't tell him the truth that having a normal test result doesn't guarantee anything. Joe is so scared he can't hear that all invasive and even minimally invasive tests come with risks of serious complications. He can't possibly hear when the doctor rattles off the standard and greatly minimized warnings, "risk of perforation, infection, and even death." Joe is so afraid he might have undiscovered cancer he will do anything for his peace of mind— even if it does jeopardize his life.

After all the testing is done, Joe's doctor doesn't find anything abnormal or in need of treatment. The insurance claim form ICD-9 code is for simple gastritis and the CPT codes are many—upper endoscopy, gastroscopy, biopsies of the esophagus and stomach, cultures of the stomach, just to name a few. Of course, after all that testing, the gastroenterologist can't just send Joe home empty-handed, so she dashes off a prescription for Nexium, the famous "little purple pill" you've seen advertised on television. Nexium is a medication called a proton pump inhibitor, which will help decrease the amount of acid in Joe's stomach and may help with his heartburn. She doesn't bother to tell Joe the potential side effects, everything from diarrhea, constipation, and muscle pains to—at the extreme—heart attacks, blood clots, and even death. But she does cheerfully inform him that he'll probably have to be on that medication indefinitely. Joe doesn't mind. After all, the co-pay is low and he's getting what he believes is a magic pill. And he doesn't have cancer. What's there to complain about?

YOUR BODY ISN'T A NUMBER ON A FORM

How could this story have gone differently? For Joe's part, he could have not reacted so quickly to the symptom of heartburn and taken the story of the young man who died of stomach cancer personally. After all the man had nothing to do with Joe. Joe would have been much better off if he just waited and didn't react out of fear. Time and our beautifully engineered bodies have a miraculous way of healing if left to our own devices without introducing fear and invasive procedures at the first symptom of something wrong. In fact in my many decades of practicing medicine I learned not to react and to allow the body to dictate the best course of action before recommending an aggressive direction that holds no certainty or promise to help anything but the bottom line of the healthcare system.

How we respond to horror stories like the one Joe's friend told him is always traumatic, dramatic, and potentially dangerous. During my days in the ER, I saw hundreds of people who came through the doors with minor chest pains, terrified they were having a heart attack just because a friend or relative had recently been diagnosed with one. The more we identify with someone else's medical problem, the more likely we are to become victims of the system. When a human being is scared, he or she makes irrational decisions. When we are afraid, we feel helpless, and allow doctors who don't know us to make life-altering decisions for us. This is what is so dangerous about fear, it sends us right into the arms of a cruel and careless system designed to benefit financially from keeping us scared and victimized.

No one else lives in your body but you. No doctor ever understands how you feel. So why are you allowing anyone with an MD to run your health and life?

DOCTORS MAKE MISTAKES TOO

Don't forget, doctors are human and unfortunately, no matter how good their intentions, their own fears, needs, and egos often cloud their judgment. Ironically, Joe's internist was also scared. Imagine how different the outcome could have been had the internist openly discussed his own concerns about taking Joe's problem to the next level. What if he had just asked Joe enough questions and made some commonsense connections between his lifestyle and his symptoms? What if the doctor put the patient's well-being ahead of the "standard of care"?

Consider this alternate approach: through an honest and connected doctor-patient dialogue, the doctor and Joe evaluate Joe's diet, eliminating or adding certain foods, looking more closely at stressors in Joe's job and his home life, and consider sleep and other lifestyle factors that could be contributing to his heartburn. Then, the internist asks Joe to keep a daily journal of his diet and how he feels mentally and physically one hour, then three hours after each meal. When Joe returns for a follow up appointment a couple of weeks later, the internist reviews the diary with Joe and makes further recommendations before considering more aggressive action. If the symptoms persist, he recommends Joe try one of the many over-the-counter antacids or medications with decades of excellent safety records as a first line of treatment. The internist puts Joe's health in Joe's hands and as partners they work together to consider when, and if, a more aggressive approach is warranted. In this scenario, Joe is in charge of his health and the doctor is his partner focused solely on helping Joe make intelligent and safe decisions.

Conventional medicine stubbornly refuses to recognize the fact that most significant health improvements don't come from pills, procedures, and tests, but from the patient's ownership of their health.

Positive changes in a patient's diet, sleep, exercise, stress management, and lifestyle will invariably help improve outcome regardless of how sick the patient is. As we discussed in the previous two chapters, medical training has always emphasized disease over prevention and healthy lifestyle choices. Unless a doctor can put a label on a symptom, diagnose a disease, and prescribe a pill or a treatment, he doesn't have the interest, time or the training to investigate other potential contributing factors, or realize it is the patient's life and the patient is ultimately responsible for it. Since insurance companies have slashed fees for a regular doctor's visit, it's no longer worth the doctors' time to just talk to the patient and work out a simple, nonaggressive treatment plan. Unless the visit leads to procedures or tests that generate more money, there is no incentive to spend real time in a heart-to-heart talk with a patient.

Most doctors tell me that, with just five to ten minutes allotted per patient visit due to the number of patients a doctor needs to see to earn his/her keep, they don't have enough time to get to know the patient. I strongly disagree. I think the real reasons doctors don't look more deeply into their patients' lives is because they weren't trained to make a connection between lifestyle and health and, for the most part, they just don't care. Tragically, patients are willing accomplices in this disastrous situation. It's a lot easier to say, "I am broken and need fixing" than it is to say, "I'm going to take responsibility for my life and fix myself."

THE SHARK'S MOUTH

After almost forty years of practicing medicine, I am still baffled that so many people willingly jump into the shark's mouth, with the full knowledge and understanding of our horrifically flawed healthcare system, and why so few fight back and refuse to be consumed in the feeding frenzy.

The truth is that unless your doctor is your advocate, your partner in your health care, you don't stand a chance at getting better. So your job is twofold.

First you must take ownership of your health. No matter how great your doctor, it's your body, you live in it, and you can't allow anyone to dictate what can be done to you.

Second, eliminate fear as a motivating factor. That's the more difficult part. To reach that goal you must make medical decisions based solely on carefully considered, honest information that is relevant to your situation. Sometimes this is very hard to accomplish because there are so many different sources of information and they all have their own agenda. You have to personally figure out where you are philosophically when it comes to your health. Are you someone who feels more comfortable with lots of testing? Do you feel better going to doctors for reassurance and professional opinions? Or are you someone who is clear that no matter what the tests might show, you won't allow anything invasive done to your body unless it's a matter of life or death? You must have the answers to these questions long before a real medical problem occurs. This way you can prepare for a medical encounter with a clear mind and won't have to react on the spot from a position of fear.

If you don't take the time and make the effort to understand yourself, you are likely to fall into the rabbit hole of never-ending tests, procedures, and visits to specialists leading to poor quality of life and no guarantee for cures or improvement in your condition.

One more thing; even if a test demonstrates an abnormality, don't jump to conclusions until you and your doctors have carefully made connections that make sense rather than working on assumptions or statistical data that may not apply to you.

I've seen hundreds of patients with abnormalities on their tests that never really correlate with their symptoms. When you go to the doctor with a specific complaint s/he will invariably search for a diagnosis to label you with. To get to the diagnosis most often you will be sent for a test: blood, Xray, ultrasound, CT scan, MRI. In my extensive experience, there have been many instances where the findings on these tests do not necessarily correlate with the cause of the problem and yet people are continuously treated solely on the results of tests.

For example: you have a pain in your back. You go to the doctor and after examining you the doctor sends you for an MRI because you might have a herniated disk. Indeed, the MRI shows a herniated disk in your spine at a level not exactly corresponding to the area of the pain. What do you do? Do you treat with medication and physical therapy? Do you give it some time or do you consider surgery? Too often, people rush into surgery when, in fact they would've been better served by less invasive treatments. Remember my patient, Lauren, who wound up with a cascade of issues when it all started with fatigue? I've seen many patients like Lauren, who undergo treatments and surgeries that leave them sicker than when they first went to the doctor, without ever solving the original problem. That is part of the huge healthcare problem we are facing every day; over diagnosing, over testing, and over treating.

Now take this huge problem and move it to the next level. The insurance company who is supposed to decide on the validity of the claim your doctor submits. How could an adjuster at the insurance company know what is really going on with the patient? Even with test results and documentation from the doctor there is no way to know if the patient is being treated correctly or not. Why? Because the adjuster is not a doctor and the adjustor never saw the patient! What kind of protection does this situation offer to any of us? None.

NUMBERS DON'T TELL THE REAL STORY

At fifty-five years old, ruggedly handsome Liam looked pale, tired and drawn. A former construction foreman who'd worked his way to managing his own general contracting business, he came to see me complaining of loss of libido, inability to build muscle, general malaise, and mild depression. I did my usual intake for a new patient; took an extensive history and spent as much time as he needed to get a comprehensive understanding of his life. After the intake we decided to do blood work. Liam's results failed to show anything out of the ordinary. His PSA was normal and his testosterone, according to guidelines set by the American Academy of Urology, was on the lower tertile (1/3) of the normal range. Since his testosterone levels had never been checked before his initial visit with me, we had no way of knowing what Liam's normal testosterone levels were before he started feeling lousy. I formed my initial opinion based on information I gathered from Liam, decided to ignore the results of the blood tests because they did not fit the clinical picture of the man standing in front of me, and using my twenty-five plus year experience with hormone therapies in patients presenting with similar symptoms, I prescribed testosterone in physiologic (low doses not to exceed normal testosterone levels in a forty-five year old) doses in a gel form his local drugstore would fill. I also spent time providing Liam with guidelines for lifestyle changes to help him manage his stress, and told him to come back in six weeks so we could check on how he was doing. This is what I call a commonsense diagnosis based on patient history and my extensive experience in the field. It is not a protocol. I am not a urologist. I'm an internist who focuses on prevention, so my diagnoses are made in partnership with my patients and the goal is to improve the quality of life with the lowest possible doses of hormones, supplements and medications. Also, lifestyle, diet, exercise, sleep, stress management always are part of the prescription for my patients.

Happily, Liam thrived on the testosterone and the lifestyle recommendations. All his symptoms and complaints disappeared and his *general health dramatically improved. As his depression lifted, he started working out again and building muscle. He also made a point of eating healthier foods and making sure he got enough sleep every night to help compensate for his stressful job. What made Liam the happiest was that his sex drive had returned! Most significantly, the very basic and small yet crucial lifestyle changes he had made quickly turned into lifelong habits.*

For the next ten years, with little more than a tweak of his testosterone levels and some supplements to help build his immune system and decrease inflammation, Liam was a model of perfect health. When he turned sixty, he went for a cardiac workup, which prompted his cardiologist to enthusiastically proclaim, "You have the heart of a thirty-five-year-old!"

Then, shortly after Liam's sixty-fifth birthday, his insurance company suddenly announced it would no longer pay for his testosterone prescription. The decision seemed bizarre and arbitrary. Liam wasn't exactly a financial drain on the insurance company. He wasn't on any other medication—which is statistically extraordinary for a man of his age—and he did not go from specialist to specialist for interminable tests. Liam was on the phone with the insurance claims representative for days on end. Arguing, reasoning, pleading, and begging didn't help. The insurance company representatives wouldn't budge.

Finally, our office got involved. The insurance company demanded we produce Liam's test results for the previous ten years. After we sent in the results, they informed us that Liam should never have been placed on testosterone in the first place because his initial lab values were within "normal" range according to their protocols.

Just when all seemed lost, a sympathetic clerk at the insurance company came to our rescue. She told me "off the record" that the company demanded its claims clerks deny all initial claims and that because of his test numbers, Liam's case was an easy "no" for them. She suggested that I warn the company in a legal letter that if my patient's health deteriorated after the medication was discontinued, as his doctor, I would hold the company liable. That statement, the clerk said, would send the case "upstairs" to the medical board for a review.

I did exactly as she advised and within four hours, Liam's prescription for testosterone was approved. He remains on it to this day, and though I'm about to go to his seventieth birthday party, you'd never guess he's a day over forty-five.

It's your choice. Even though no one individual can fix America's healthcare mess, I believe it's up to each one of us to determine our path. You decide whether you are a victim or a survivor.

CHAPTER 4
ONE PILL TO SAVE US ALL:
PART I

"It is easy to get a thousand prescriptions but hard to get one single remedy."

—Chinese Proverb

One day, back when I was in charge of a busy ER, I was called by one of the residents to help with a patient. He was bleeding from his stomach and no one could figure out why. The patient was a healthy young man in his twenties with no history of stomach problems or other medical issues. In fact, he was an amateur athlete and had completed a 10K run that very morning. As an ER doctor, you always try to connect the dots—but in this guy's case, there were no dots to connect! We paged the gastroenterology fellow and while waiting for him to arrive we placed an NG (nasogastric) tube through his nose into his stomach and were lavageing (washing out) his stomach. Blood was initially coming out but the fluid aspirated quickly and turned clear with the saline solution we placed into the stomach. This meant the bleeding wasn't that serious. The resident whispered to me that maybe this guy had taken too much Motrin. There was no record of any medication on the chart so I thought that seemed an unlikely explanation, but it was worth pursuing. I went back to the bedside and spoke with the patient. He admitted that yes, he had been taking Motrin. He suffered a sprained ankle two weeks before and with the 10K coming up, hadn't wanted to take time off from training. First, he said, he took Motrin for the pain, but then a friend told him to take Aleve because it was much better, so he decided to add it to the Motrin. When his mother told him that Ibuprofen was the only painkiller to trust, he added that to the mix, as well. In short order, he was taking all these non-steroidal anti-inflammatories (NSAIDs) to the tune of twenty pills a day! He had neglected to mention this when he was admitted because they were over-the-counter medications, which he said "didn't count." The poor guy never realized they were all exactly the same drug—ibuprofen— and that he was suffering the side effects of an overdose of NSAIDs.

OVER THE COUNTER CURE-ALLS

Over-the-counter (OTC) medications are dangerous, but physicians almost never talk about them. Many of these drugs start out as prescription medications, but once their patents run out, the dosing changes and they get moved into the OTC market. Medical school doesn't include training in OTC medication so doctors know very little about them. Because they are available without a prescription, patients believe these drugs are innocuous and it rarely occurs to them to mention them to the doctor. This leaves a huge gap in the flow of information in the area of medications. It also leaves the public with the notion that OTC medications are innocuous and are safe cure-alls we can access without a doctor's help.

I hate to ruin another fantasy for you, but there is not now, nor will there ever be, a "magic pill" that can guarantee to keep you safe and healthy.

Yet, most of us want to believe in a magic pill. And pharmaceutical companies use their considerable resources to convince us they can deliver that magic pill to you anytime now. Americans have been programmed to believe that there's always a pill to cure whatever ails us. Interestingly, in my experience, Europeans do not have the same cure-all mentality. The search for the Holy Grail in a magic pill seems to be a uniquely American concept.

When it comes to curing what ails us, why do so many Americans expect a quick fix? Perhaps it started with the American pioneers who bought into the snake oil cure-all mentality that arose during the 1700s. Self-proclaimed "doctors" with no more medical credentials than a barber would travel the countryside, selling all kinds of elixirs and potions with claims they could cure an improbable litany of ailments. These salespeople were usually mesmerizing and gifted orators and it was hard not to become ensnared by their convincing presentations. By the time customers discovered it was all hype, the "doctor" was long gone. Not much has changed in the last three hundred years. Today, we still buy into infomercials with their promise of better bodies, thicker hair, and longer-lasting erections.

It could also be the lingering myth of American exceptionalism—the idea that we are the greatest, smartest, richest, and most technologically advanced country in the world. If we believe this, then of course it follows that we must be able to produce a pill to fix everything. I use the word "myth" for a reason—it is just that. It's hard for me to understand how politicians can still declare "We have the best medical system in the world!" when America's health statistics consistently tell a very different story. We are living in the middle of the most monumental healthcare disaster ever. The United States spends more than twice as much per person on healthcare as any other industrial nation, yet according to the Johns Hopkins Bloomberg School of Public Health, the health of Americans overall is ranked second to last.[25] While we cling to the possibility that all the "medical breakthroughs" we read about will protect us from our own mortality, according to John's Hopkins School of Public Health, "On most [health] indicators, the U.S. relative performance declined since 1960; not one of the measured variables improved."[26]

Snake oil is still being sold to the American public and the circus isn't leaving town any time soon. Those magic elixir salesmen of yesteryear are today's pharmaceutical mega corporations, and the media are their carnival barkers.

There are lots of winners when we perpetuate the snake oil mentality. Above all, the pharmaceutical corporations and their partners: hospitals, academic institutions and the research they sponsor, politicians they pay for, and advertising and marketing companies that produce and distribute their ads. Not to mention media that gets paid hundreds of millions of dollars to air their ads. Drug companies have at their disposal the strongest sales force in the U.S.; thousands of lawyers in hundreds of legal firms, dealing with regulatory aspects of the industry and class action suits arising from side effects of their drugs; and last, but not least, more than seven hundred thousand doctors in the trenches.

WHAT YOUR DOCTOR WILL NEVER TELL YOU: THE WORLD OF OTC

You can't convince people to buy a magic pill unless you first convince them they have a problem that needs fixing. I had a friend who was a pharmaceutical advertising maven during the first decade of the 21st century. The information he gave me was priceless. He told me in no uncertain terms that, "You have to create the need. Patients don't know they need a medication. You have to tell them they have a problem that your medication will solve." Even if you don't feel sick enough to go to a doctor, pharmaceutical companies will figure out how to sell you medication you don't even know you need. You can just go to one of the ever-expanding drugstore chains whose shelves are stocked aisle after aisle with medications to treat the common cold, diarrhea, constipation, congestion, allergies, headache, heartburn, belly aches, poison ivy, and itchy skin…you name it, there's a remedy for it.

In theory, people like me, who encourage patients to take charge of their own health, support the idea of OTC medicines because they don't require a doctor's prescription. If you take responsibility for your own health, you don't need to run to the doctor every time you have a sniffle. OTC medications are there to help. In fact, in Europe the OTC industry includes antibiotics, sedatives and many other medications we can only get by prescription in the U.S. Are people smarter in Europe? Maybe they just take more responsibility for their lives and health than we do.

OTC is a massively profitable business. In 2014, according to the Consumer Healthcare Products Association[27] total spending on non-prescription health products was $31 billion. That's a pretty hefty number. Let's go back to those well-stocked aisles at your local CVS, Walgreen's, Duane Reade or Rite Aid. Stroll over to the "pain relief" aisle and count the number of choices you have. Is your head spinning yet? Most consumers will flash back to a convincing commercial they've seen, perhaps one extoling the virtues of Aleve over Advil (invariably produced by Aleve). "Aleve is the best," the consumer will decide, even though it's priced higher than the store's generic NSAID, even though they both have exactly the same active ingredient in the same dose: ibuprofen. Advil has its own convincing commercial that another customer will remember and just like the first customer, she'd rather pay extra money for the "best" brand rather than save considerably on a generic. The competition for customer loyalty is a big business, which has little to do with the quality or effectiveness of OTC drugs.

Although there are hundreds of brands and packages, it's all marketing smoke and mirrors. There are very few differences between non-steroidal anti-inflammatories. Ibuprofen is the active medication in every NSAID. Motrin, Aleve, Ibuprofen, Advil are just different labels for the same product. The same goes for OTC cold and allergy medications. There is little or no distinction in their active ingredients, yet advertising companies work overtime to convince you that one is better than the other.

Researchers at the University of Chicago Booth School of Business[28] analyzed Nielsen Homescan data that covered more than seventy-seven million shopping trips between 2004 and 2011. Medical professionals (doctors and pharmacists) were more likely to buy generic headache remedies than brand names when compared to their nonmedical peers. That's because they know ibuprofen by any other name is just ibuprofen. Since this was a business school study, the researchers were interested in consumer behavior. What they found should terrify brand-name OTC companies: statistically, if consumers knew as much about their headache meds as their doctors or pharmacists (89 percent of who are more likely to be familiar with the active ingredients than the average consumer) they would opt for generics. According to the study, a change in consumer awareness could cause the brand-name medication companies to lose a whopping 55 percent of their sales, costing them about $410 million dollars in profits. It's no wonder OTC companies want to keep you in the dark about the importance of reading the ingredients on the label.

The potential danger of this ignorance is that you can easily take many times the recommended dosage if you buy more than one OTC med just like the young man at the beginning of this chapter did. Another example: if you have the flu you might take a pain reliever for body aches and a cold pill for the sniffles. Without reading the label, you won't realize that the cold pill actually has twice the amount of the same active ingredient as the pain reliever. Since doctors have no training in OTCs, they too discount them as harmless and not strong enough to make a difference. That's why doctors seldom consider what (or how many) OTC drugs their patient is taking when writing a prescription. Many doctors will unwittingly give a patient the same drug in prescription strength that s/he is quietly taking at home, leading to an increased chance of overdose or serious side effects.

THERE IS NO FREE LUNCH AND THERE'S NO CONSEQUENCE-FREE PILL

It's vital you never forget that every pill you take—whether a vitamin, painkiller, antibiotic, cough medicine, or supplement—will always affect you and will interact with everything else you take, eat, or drink. A study published in the *Journal of American Medicine* (JAMA) looked at the differences in advertising between four products (Schering-Plough's Claritin or loratidine and AstraZeneca's Prilosec or omeprazole; Glaxo Smith Kline's Alli or orlistat and McNeil's Zyrtec or cetirizine), comparing them while they were still prescription and afterward, when they went OTC. What they found is both interesting and quite scary—presentation of the drugs' benefits went up after the switch to OTC (from 83 percent to 97 percent), while the presentation of the drug's potential harms or side effects shockingly dropped like a lead balloon (from 70 percent to just 11 percent). "With the exception of print advertisements for orlistat, no post-switch advertisements mentioned contra-indications or adverse effects," wrote the study's authors. That's because once a drug becomes available over the counter, it moves from being regulated by the FDA (Federal Drug Administration) to the FTC (Federal Trade Commission). The FTC has lower standards of "truthfulness" in labeling and does not require balance between potential benefits and harms. Thus, the OTC drug manufacturing companies have no mandate to warn you or your doctor (except in the tiny fine print on the label) about potential harmful side effects. Here are a few of the most egregious examples:

1. **ACETAMINOPHEN (Tylenol)**

   Each year, acetaminophen overdose is responsible for more than 56,000 emergency room visits, 2,600 hospitalizations, and an estimated 458 deaths due to acute liver failure. In fact, just taking one or two pills above the recommended dosage for two weeks or more can be deadlier than a one-time Tylenol overdose.

2. **OTC LAXATIVES (sodium phosphate laxatives)**

   Can cause dehydration or abnormal levels of electrolytes in the blood, leading to kidney damage even at recommended doses. Most at risk are young children, adults over fifty-five, and patients using other medications (and don't forget — everyone does) that may affect kidney function.

3. **COUGH AND COLD MEDICINES**

   Dextromethorphan, an ingredient in all cough and many cold remedies that was created as an alternative to codeine, can be dangerous and deadly if taken in higher than recommended amounts and can lead to impaired judgment, euphoria, dizziness, loss of coordination, nausea and vomiting, hallucinations, respiratory depression, coma, and death.

4. **ASPIRIN**

   The NIH (National Institutes of Health) has recently warned doctors to scale back on recommending patients take a daily baby aspirin as a heart attack or stroke preventive. In people who don't have significant risk factors for heart attack or stroke, a daily aspirin—even at low doses—can cause bleeding in the gastrointestinal tract and even in the brain.

   "Pharmaceuticals do not lose their ability of harm after moving from behind the pharmacist's counter to in front of it; misuse of OTC drugs remains a major cause of emergency department visits, hospitalization and death," wrote the authors of the *JAMA* study, four of whom were at Brigham and William's Hospital in Boston, the fifth who worked for CVS Caremark. The study's lead author, Dr. Jeremy Greene, is now at John's Hopkins University, which strongly emphasizes consumer and patient rights and safety.

Unfortunately, many of these crucial warnings may be off your doctor's radar and that can have tragic consequences—sometimes, even for doctors themselves.

A NOT-SO-HAPPY ANNIVERSARY

They had just come back from celebrating their twenty-fifth anniversary. He was fifty-five, she was fifty. They were as much in love as they had been on their wedding day—in fact, much more so.

He was a physician, she a nurse. They were in training in the same hospital when they first saw each other. It was, as the French say, "un coup de foudre"—a bolt of lightning. He immediately lost himself in her deep, hypnotic brown eyes and she was mesmerized by his calm strength and easy way of dealing with the world. Almost instantly, they became a couple and their devotion to one another took hold. They were married within a year.

The decades passed all too quickly. He became a prominent cardiologist. They had four children and she stayed home for a few years, tending to their growing brood. When the kids left for college, she went back to the hospital working on the medical service that she always loved. They also started to travel together. Neither had any serious medical problems and they were both diligent about their annual physicals—she about her mammograms, both about their colonoscopies, and they even made sure to take some of the less common tests, like stress tests to rule out heart problems. Together, they took long brisk walks every day for exercise. They lived the good life, which as they traveled more, began to include eating gourmet, often heavy, foods and drinking plenty of excellent wines. As a cardiologist, he wasn't worried, since their general health was so good, but he decided he would add another layer of protection by taking a baby aspirin every day and a statin to keep his cholesterol from getting too high. They both felt that this way, there was a lot more room for error when it came to their increasing indulgences. He felt protected. They grew closer over the years. Their older kids were parents now, and grandparenting was another magical pleasure that filled the couple's charmed lives with joy. As they reached their twenty-fifth year together the future looked bright and full of promise.

They took a luxury cruise to celebrate their anniversary—and celebrate they most certainly did. For an entire week on the opulent ocean liner, they ate and drank to their heart's content. They sipped fruity cocktails by the pool, danced late into the night, and were invited to sit at the captain's table. When their children and grandchildren met them at the dock, everyone agreed that their parents literally glowed with happiness and love.

Their first night back home, in the rush to unpack and settle back in, the cardiologist was running up and down the stairs of their home when he tripped and fell, hitting his head against the carved mahogany banister. He said it was just a bump, nothing that a little ice wouldn't fix. She brought him the ice and he held it to his head for a few minutes until the pain subsided. Then they both resumed unpacking without another thought. Since the next day was a workday, they turned in before midnight with their arms wrapped around each other, satisfied and grateful for their beautiful life together.

The next morning, she was awakened not by the alarm, but by her husband's snoring. He had always been a snorer, but this was far louder than what she was used to hearing. As she had done hundreds of times before, she tried to gently shake him awake. Oddly, he didn't respond. She decided he must have been exhausted from the trip, so she got out of bed and started her morning routine. The alarm clock sounded about a half hour later. When the buzzing didn't stop, she went back to the bedroom to make sure he was up because she knew he had an early consultation. To her surprise, he was still asleep, and when she shook him hard, he still didn't wake up.

At this point, she switched from wife to nurse mode and began an evaluation of her husband. There was no sign of anything wrong. His breathing was normal, his pulse regular. His heart sounded normal as well. She brought her blood pressure cuff into the bedroom and his blood pressure albeit borderline—130/86—was fairly normal, too. What was wrong with him? She called 911. When the paramedics arrived, they had no diagnosis that made sense. They gave him oxygen in his nose and took him out on a stretcher and on to the hospital.

Once at the hospital where they both worked, the cardiologist got VIP treatment. All their friends and colleagues from different specialties and departments converged on the ER to see him and offer their own advice. But they too were stumped. His heart was fine, vital signs fine, neurologic exam normal—except he wouldn't wake up. As the doctors gathered around his bed trying to agree on their next step, the cardiologist opened his eyes. Confused, he sat up in bed and asked them what he was doing in the ER. When they told him, he laughed and said they were all crazy. After gently chiding his wife for overreacting, he jumped off the stretcher and hurried off to his office hours. He admitted to his friend, a neurologist that he had a bit of a headache and promised he'd check in if it got worse. Both agreed it was probably from sleeping too much.

The day proceeded as normally as any other. He saw his patients, went to lunch with a friend, played a vigorous round of tennis, and then went back to the hospital to check on his patients before going home for dinner. His headache had worsened a bit, but he didn't bother to call the neurologist because he decided it must be dehydration from the tennis game.

When he got home, his wife was waiting anxiously with a big glass of wine and a home-cooked meal: pasta with marinara sauce and lamb chops, his favorites. She was disappointed when he told her he wasn't really up for dinner because of the headache, and that he'd probably overdone it at tennis that day and was exhausted. He took a couple of Advil, his usual baby aspirin, and went to bed early.

He never woke up again.

His autopsy report showed a massive subdural hematoma (blood clot under the main covering of the brain) caused by the blow to his head, which had spread over a larger area during the course of the day prior to his death. On its own the initial subdural bleed might not have killed him. But there was a large amount of bleeding that continued over the course of the day that became deadly. It is very likely the further bleeding was caused by a side-effect of the baby aspirin he took for over a decade to prevent a heart attack.

I don't really blame doctors for their lack of knowledge and disregard for OTC medications. I do blame the pharmaceutical marketing machines. They won't stop trying to sell so it's high time we, the general public, take responsibility for improving the situation. We must all understand that every medication we take has side effects. No matter how benign or safe it is promoted to be, it can turn deadly on a dime. And deadly can only happen once.

THE MEGA-MARKETING OF DRUGSTORES

The small town pharmacy is an endangered species in America. A handful of mega drugstore chains have taken over not only the sale of OTC medications, but also the dispensing of prescriptions. Cheaper prices, a wide variety of products, and convenience are the main reasons for their success. A mega pharmacy has a full complement of OTC drugs, makeup, hair care and cosmetic products, body creams, dental supplies, disposable cameras and photograph or digital printing, pantyhose, underwear, sweatshirts, household and personal care appliances, hardware, cleaning supplies, stationery, plants, home décor items, last-minute gifts, greeting cards, and even groceries. Your local mega pharmacy will even sell you canned, boxed, and bottled food. And their vendors subsidize their advertising budgets. The dollars they spend on ads is staggering. For example, according to the data center of *Ad Age Magazine* in 2010, Walgreen Company disclosed net ad costs of $271 million, but it also received $197 million in advertising allowances from vendors[29]. This means that Walgreens poured a total of $468 million into advertising that year—$271 million from its own coffers and the rest put up by suppliers. Vendor allowances accounted for 42 percent of Walgreen's gross ad costs in 2010. That's a powerful advertising machine to be reckoned with.

DRIVE-THRU HEALTH CARE

The latest and even more lucrative trend in these mega pharmacies is to become one-stop shops for medical advice and even minor emergency care[30]. Following the successful model of CVS, a market pioneer, other drugstore chains are opening walk-in clinics inside the store next to their pharmacies. *Atlantic Magazine* reported in 2014 that there were around 1,700 walk-in medical clinics across the country in drug and big-box stores and supermarkets, like CVS, Walgreens, Target, and Kroger, increasing at a rate of about 20 percent per year[31]. They're spreading like wildfire across the country, staffed by nurses and physician's assistants these makeshift operations offer basic medical services, including diagnosis and treatment of common infections, vaccinations, treatment for minor injuries, and routine lab tests at usually under $99. Currently, Walmart has a plan to corner the market by charging $40 for a simple visit and $8 for a basic lab test.

On the surface, this trend seems like it could be a potentially positive development[32], empowering consumers to get health care for minor problems without long waits or delayed appointments. This is,something that, in theory, I support. Patients can skip the lengthy wait at a hospital ER or their doctor's office, get in and out quickly and cheaply, and even have the convenience to get some other shopping done while they wait for their prescriptions to get filled. Already more than twenty million people have been treated in these walk-in pharmacy clinics since their inception and the numbers are growing.

However, as with the rest of the fast and furious façade of modern medicine in America, you've got to follow the money trail to get the real story. Having an in-pharmacy medical clinic to provide medical care and prescribe medications seems logical. Prescriptions generated by the clinic, will immediately be filled by the in-house pharmacy. How ingenious. One stop shopping that keeps business in-house. Once there is the ability to prescribe medications inside the store, the patient is captive audience and is unlikely to take the prescription to another pharmacy.

INSTANT HEALTH FOR SALE

A patient and friend told me a particularly disturbing story about her college-age daughter, Sara, and her late-night encounter with a pharmacy walk-in clinic. After a wild weekend of parties at her sorority, Sara was feeling crummy. She thought it was more than the usual hangover, so she went to the college health services. The nurse on-call examined her and diagnosed a mild respiratory virus that was going around campus. She recommended a couple days of rest, hydration, and no alcohol. She told her the virus usually lasted twenty-four to forty-eight hours.

Sara didn't want a virus to interfere with her busy social life. There was a big party on campus that weekend she didn't want to miss, so she decided to go to the local Walgreens to get some Advil and a decongestant to at least get rid of some of the symptoms. While she was roaming the "Cold and Flu" aisle, trying to make sense of the labels on the medications, a friendly salesperson approached her. She told Sara that if she needed medical help there was a doctor on the premises, who could see her right away, right there in the store. There was no wait and within a few minutes, a nurse practitioner invited Sara into a makeshift office at the back of the store. After five minutes of listening to Sara's description of the problem, the nurse told her she was going to give her an antibiotic to "speed up the recovery process" and a prescription-strength painkiller for her body aches. The woman turned to her computer and told Sara she could go up to the pharmacy counter and pick up her prescription in ten minutes. She also raved about a new brand of makeup that just came into the store and recommended Sara check it out while she was waiting. "I just bought some myself and love it." Sara ended up leaving Walgreens with two prescriptions, ibuprofen, decongestants and about fifty dollars' worth of makeup.

It's not clear whether the nurse practitioner was there to provide medical care or sell products. Antibiotics do not treat viruses and, in general, it is not wise to hand out prescription painkillers to college students. Fortunately, Sara didn't take the medications and as the campus nurse had predicted, she was soon better. However, the reason she didn't take the antibiotics was because she wanted to drink, not because she doubted the nurse. This story is a rather sad commentary on our healthcare system. Placing a licensed professional in a pharmacy so that more prescriptions can be written and filled in the same place seems to me a blatant sales strategy, not a shred of care for the health of the public.

I have serious concerns about the trend walk-in drugstore "clinics" are setting. I see them as further proof of the dangers inherent to the move away from personal relationship-based medicine to a profit-based, anonymous, one-size-fits-all type of care that takes further advantage of people's fears and desire for a quick fix regardless of who or how it is delivered. Would you really want to have a powerful pharmaceutical prescribed to you or your children by a total stranger? Walk-in pharmacy clinics are nothing more than storefronts set up to keep business in the pharmacy. They don't care about you; they only care about their bottom line.

If you want to get the kind of health care that will realistically protect you, you need someone who knows and cares about you. And when it comes to prescription medications, the situation is even more dire.

CHAPTER 5
ONE PILL TO SAVE US ALL:
PART II

"To live by medicine is to live horribly."

—Carolus Linnaeus

YOUR DOCTOR AND BIG PHARMA

When it comes to the dangers and controversies surrounding OTC drugs, let's agree to cut your doctor some slack. His or her negligence in failing to steer you away from the risks and dangers of OTC medicines almost always arises from ignorance and inadequate medical education.

However, if your physician has too cozy a relationship with any of the huge pharmaceutical companies, their products, and their salespeople, that's another story altogether. Since the early 2000s, the FDA has cracked down hard on all the perks pharmaceutical companies were offering to physicians and their families in the '80s and '90s in exchange for endorsement (writing prescriptions) for their medications:, luxury all-expense-paid vacations, junkets, and highly valuable gifts. Today, drug companies are limited by very strict rules. They can barely buy a doctor who prescribes their medications a 'reasonably' priced office lunch for the staff. But these mega corporations, known as "Big Pharma," still have powerful influence over the prescribing practices of doctors. As a former acquaintance of mine, who was a high-powered adman for the pharmaceutical industry, once cynically told me, "The drug companies consider all you doctors as their unpaid salespeople."

The power big pharmaceutical companies have over American healthcare policy cannot be overstated—from their coercive influence at the governmental level, to their input into medical school curriculum, to the employment practices of the FDA, to their ownership of a majority of health care (including insurance companies), to their direct influence on doctors and patients. Here are a few—just the tip of the iceberg—of the most stunning facts[33]:

Every year, pharmaceutical corporations are at the top of the Fortune 500 list—the most profitable businesses in the world. Four of them are headquartered in the U.S.: Johnson & Johnson (#39), Pfizer (#51), Merck (#65), and Eli Lilly (#129).

The median revenue of the top pharmaceutical companies in 2013-2014 was $95.1 billion.

The top eleven companies generated nearly three quarters of a TRILLION dollars in pure profit in just one decade.

Big Pharma outspends all other industries in lobbying the U.S. government and the FDA. From 1998 to 2013, it spent $2.7 BILLION in lobbying, 42 percent more than the second-highest lobbying big spender (which was...you guessed it... the insurance industry!).

As the pharma-insurance influence on Obamacare I noted in Chapter 3 clearly demonstrates, our government is bought, paid for, and brought to you by the biggest gorillas in the room: Big Pharma and big insurance.

UNCLE PHARMA WANTS YOU!

Many decades ago, federal regulations made advertising prescription drugs directly to the public illegal so drug companies focused on marketing their medications to doctors, clinics and hospitals. In those days doctors couldn't advertise either so it was all about location and word of mouth. Today, they're coming after you directly.

Before the late 1990s, when there was no direct-to-consumer advertising of prescription drugs on television, in magazines, or on the Internet, the average patient had no knowledge of what brand-name or generic medications were available, nor were consumers conversant in the names of hundreds of diseases and conditions. When a doctor wrote a prescription, he would tell the patient how often to take the medication, what it might interact with, what it was supposed to do, and what side effects to look out for. This was part of the doctor-patient interaction.

If a patient wanted to know more there was one way to find out: the omnipresent PDR (*Physician's Desk Reference*) that some consumers and all doctors had in their libraries. And, while some did read the PDR, most relied on their relationship with the doctor.

Today, the average American television viewer is inundated with as many as nine prescription drug ads per day—a total of sixteen hours of ads per year.[34] It concerns me that those sixteen hours spent watching slickly-produced ads for cure-all pills are far more time than the average person spends with his or her primary care physician in any given year.

MASS MEDIA AND MAGIC PILLS

Beginning in the early 1980s (is it a coincidence that this is the same period when insurance companies also began their climb to monopoly?) the Federal Drug Administration (FDA)—the branch of the U.S. government tasked with protecting consumers by monitoring the safety and licensing of drugs—began to gradually relax its rules for advertising and marketing prescription medications. As the powerful lobbyists of big pharmaceutical companies descended on Washington D.C. and began to throw some of their billions around, the previous rules that demanded strict and rigorous listings of both the benefits and dangers of every drug marketed to physicians and the public became looser and looser. By 1997, the FDA had opened the floodgates for pharmaceutical companies—not just to continue to market their name-brand prescription medications to doctors, but to be able to hawk their miracle cures to the average Joe and Jane, sitting at home on their sofas watching TV. The carnival barkers and snake oil salesmen of old returned to America in the late 20ᵗʰ Century, only now they have all the tools of modern advertising at their disposal: detailed consumer research, high-quality creative direction, cinematography, music, scriptwriting, and prime time slots on TV that allow them to zero in on exactly the right type of customer for their particular drug. If the doctors aren't going to prescribe enough of their newest, most lucrative miracle drugs, they will convince the patients to demand them.

You've seen the ads: the gauzy, dreary image of a sad woman, gazing hopelessly out the window at the pouring rain, that suddenly transforms into a smiling, happy woman in a bright, sunlit day as she runs through a field with her dog after taking THE anti-depressant; a young woman in tight, white jeans, dancing without a care because she can now take a birth control pill that insures she doesn't have to have the worry of a monthly period anymore; a model-perfect, grey-haired couple looking tired, distant and sad who, after the introduction of a magical pill to eliminate erectile dysfunction, are suddenly riding their bikes by the beach with satisfied smiles on their faces.

This strategy works—and it works brilliantly. Drug companies will argue, quite convincingly, that direct-to-consumer (DTC) ads are a giant victory for freedom of speech and freedom of information in America. They empower the consumer with information they can use to demand from their doctors all the "ground breaking" medications that are out there to save them, but need a doctor's prescription. But there's also a lot of evidence to the contrary[35]:

- DTC ads manufacture diseases and encourage drug overuse. If you didn't feel old or inadequate before you saw that Viagra ad, drug company marketing departments sure hope you will after. DTC ads contribute to the "medicalization" of normal conditions, cosmetic, issues, and trivial ailments, which ultimately lead to an overmedicated and constantly sick society.[36]

- DTC ads misinform patients by pushing their drug as the cure, while never mentioning or questioning issues of lifestyle or other possible causes for their ailments. One study showed that only 19 percent of ads reviewed mentioned lifestyle factors at all.[37]

- DTC ads overemphasize drug benefits and underplay risks. Have you ever noticed how all DTC television commercials spend most of their time on beautiful images and glowing descriptions of the benefits of their drugs, but then actually speed up when the narrator's voice lists their extensive side effects? What's more, these side effects (including risk of coma and death) are read in a monotone, barely audible voice mismatched against a backdrop of happy, peaceful, inspiring images? That's no accident. Advertisers know that when visual and verbal messages are in conflict, the visual influence on the viewer is almost always more powerful.[38] Studies have shown that once a viewer has bought into the over-the-top, seductive 'benefits' promised by the ad, he or she may ignore the risk section altogether.[39]

- DTC ads push doctors into inappropriate prescribing. If an ad convinces a patient its brand-name drug will "fix" his/her problem, s/he is likely to pressure a doctor to prescribe it. Some patients may even make up symptoms or withhold information from their doctor to fit into a particular profile for the drug they saw in a DTC ad.[40] Many doctors—either because of patient misinformation or a desire to please the patient—will just write the script, regardless of need.

So what is this doing to the already deteriorating doctor-patient relationship in America? Ask Dr. John Abramson, author of *Overdosed America:*

Increasingly, my patients were looking to pills to keep them well instead of making the changes in their own lives that evidence showed to be far more beneficial. Engaging patients in constructive dialogue about their health risks and habits—a big part of what I think is good doctoring—was becoming more difficult and occasionally impossible. Too many visits were turning into non-productive contests of wills.[41]

Like so many of my colleagues, Dr. Abramson found that suddenly his patients were coming to him convinced that their symptoms fit exactly the many new "diseases" described in these ads and were determined to get him to prescribe those magical 'breakthrough' brand-name pills. Only brand name pills would do—after all, who can resist the dreamy smiles on the faces of the actors in all those slick commercials?

Flooding the market with high-end ads for prescription drugs has turned out to be a huge financial boon for pharmaceutical companies and media who air and carry them. This is just one more way in which the drug companies have taken over the healthcare system, turning doctors into pawns in this very dangerous game.

SCIENCE? OR PROPAGANDA?

In order to maintain hospital privileges and keep licenses current, every doctor practicing in the U.S. is required to take CME (continuing medical education) courses. The courses are given in person and online by a multitude of institutions and they are accredited by Accreditation Council for Medical Education. In addition, there are hundreds of medical journals and online sites that publish research and clinical articles. The most trusted are "peer-reviewed journals" whose contents are reviewed by a panel of experts in the field covered by the article, research or information provided to establish its credibility. The *New England Journal of Medicine, Journal of the American Medical Association*, and a few others are the recognized leaders in the field, and there are hundreds specific to individual medical specialties, some peer reviewed, others not. Every specialty has its own peer-reviewed journal. Urologists have the *American Journal of Urology*, ob-gyns the *American Journal of Obstetrics and Gynecology*, surgeons the *American Journal of Surgery*, and so on. They consistently represent the opinions of the leadership in the particular specialty as promulgated by their societies. One caveat: many, if not most, "opinion leaders" and societies have deep "relationships" with pharmaceutical corporations.

What the patient doesn't know—and what many doctors don't realize—is the enormous influence that pharmaceutical companies (as well as medical equipment and instruments companies) have on the content of the "scientific research" data contained in these journals. In researching his book, *Overdosed in America*, Dr. John Abramson was stunned to discover the extent to which medical research was overseen and controlled by forces motivated solely by profit, without regard for science or patients:

"There has been a virtual takeover of medical knowledge in the United States, leaving doctors and patients little opportunity to know the truth about good medical care and no safe alternative but to pay up and go along."

KILLER PERSUASION—THE VIOXX CASE

There are many cases I can write about with the case of Premarin—the Women's Health Initiative study—as the perfect example of how conflict of interest in big pharma permeates our entire system and alters the course of health care negatively for millions. However, I made the decision to not write about it in this book because my position on hormones is known and I have written books, articles, given talks, and even lobbied Congress on that topic for more than fourteen years.

Instead I chose the classic case of Vioxx. The perfect example of Big Pharma using flawed and cherry-picked studies to sell the now infamous Vioxx and Celebrex, two prescription non-steroidal anti-inflammatories, created by Merck and Pfizer respectively to compete with the far cheaper OTC anti-inflammatories that we discussed in the last chapter—ibuprofen—labeled the likes of Motrin, Naproxen and Advil.

In the early 1990s, Merck started working on a non-steroidal anti-inflammatory drug called rofecoxib. A big problem with NSAIDs—like with the popular, and far less expensive, OTC ibuprofen, Naproxen—was that they cause stomach upset. A significant percentage of people with chronic pain who take Naproxen will develop digestive problems, including gastritis, irritation, pain, heartburn, serious bleeding, and ulcers. The drug company's marketing department recognized this was a huge problem in the NSAID market. If they could come up with a NSAID with fewer gastrointestinal side effects, the drug company would become the market leader overnight.

Merck pharmaceuticals decided it could turn Vioxx (rofecoxib) into a "blockbuster" drug if they could prove it had fewer gastrointestinal side effects than the others. To help secure the outcome, Merck sponsored a study—VIGOR (Vioxx Gastrointestinal Research Trial), which persuasively demonstrated that Vioxx users experienced fewer gastrointestinal symptoms than those taking over-the-counter NSAIDs. When Merck started trials for Vioxx, they had to get permission from the FDA to conduct human trials, which are reviewed periodically by DSMB (Data and Safety Monitoring Board) following stringent guidelines. The protocols for the clinical trials on Vioxx gastrointestinal outcomes were developed in January 1999 and initial results were reported to DSMB in October of 1999, showing several cardio-pulmonary deaths. The DSMB oddly reported that, "nothing appeared abnormal or triggered concern."[42]

Strangely, the trials continued and the FDA and DSMB never raised any questions about the deaths allowing the study to come to a positive conclusion on the frequency of gastrointestinal side effects of Vioxx. Once the data was published in the December 1999 issue of the leading peer-reviewed *JAMA* (remember, a leading peer reviewed journal in the field with unquestionable credibility), the science behind it was considered unimpeachable and the medical community, trusting the data in the study, was set up to begin prescribing this "better" drug. Merck had done the proper groundwork to establish scientific credibility and could next move on to advertising the new drug directly to consumers. Merck marketing department held a competition between top advertising companies to determine who would be the best company to promote the drug—DDB New York, FCB New York, McCann-Erickson Worldwide, and J. Walter Thompson.[43] DDB won the initial $40M contract to begin flooding the market with news of the Vioxx "breakthrough" in pain relief without the undesirable gastrointestinal side-effects of the other NSAIDs. Between 1999 and

2004, Merck spent more than $100 million in advertising and marketing to build Vioxx into one of the most popular prescription drugs of all time. Patients rushed to their doctors' offices, demanding they prescribe this new miracle pill, despite the fact that it was much more expensive than the various OTC brands of ibuprofen. Almost immediately, Vioxx was bringing in sales of more than $1 billion a year in the U.S. alone! [44]

Then, people started dying. Lots of them. Vioxx and Celebrex (its cousin from another drug company) were both linked to an increasing number of heart attacks and cardiovascular events. By September 30, 2004, when Merck removed Vioxx from the market, 60,000 people had died. Strangely the media spun the story to make the public believe that Merck had just "discovered" dangerous side effects in the drug and had "done the right thing" by taking it off the market. But the truth is much more frightening.

Back in 2000, Dr. John Abramson had read about another Merck-sponsored study on Vioxx in the *New England Journal of Medicine*. In this study, the authors attributed even greater benefits to the drug. Abramson went directly to the raw data contained in the FDA files. What he found was shocking. Although people who took Vioxx experienced twenty-one fewer serious GI complications than those who took Naproxen (its OTC counterpart), they experienced twenty-seven more serious cardiovascular complications. This crucial information had either been intentionally left out or considered statistically insignificant by the authors of the study. Abramson then checked the FDA data on Celebrex, Vioxx's competitor/cousin from Pfizer. Although Celebrex's *JAMA*-published study was longer than one year, which would ordinarily give the study more weight and credibility, it only discussed the data from the first six months of the study. Retrospectively this appears to have occurred because, as the study progressed, more complications came to light and the drug company didn't want "negative" data to "interfere" with the benefits of the drug.

"The more closely I scrutinized the data on the cardiovascular complications [of Vioxx], the more I learned about how data can be manipulated to color the 'scientific evidence' that is so trusted by the doctors and the public," wrote Abramson. [45]

As expected, there was enormous legal and legislative fallout from the Vioxx and Celebrex scandals—some of which is still ongoing today. Strangely though little of this was covered by conventional media. To find out more about what is really going on you have to go to alternative news outlets. Dr. Joseph Mercola, the author of the most popular alternative site on the Internet, blogged the following:

"Back in 2008, Dr. Joseph S. Ross of New York's Mount Sinai School of Medicine came across ghostwritten research studies for Vioxx while reviewing documents related to lawsuits filed against Merck."

It turned out the practice of using ghostwriters for scientific articles is not rare or unique. Many big pharmaceutical companies were hiring professional ghostwriters to research and write slanted interpretations of research studies to help the company they worked for. Then the companies paid "key opinion leaders"—doctors highly respected from academic institutions—to "review" the drafts and then literally sign their names as authors of the published works.

According to an April 16, 2008 article on MedHeadlines (a website dedicated to prevention and dissemination of scientific data to the public and medical profession from a non-pharmaceutical perspective):

In about 96 journal publications, Ross and his colleagues discovered internal Merck documents and e-mail messages pertaining to clinical study reports and review articles, some of which were developed by the company's marketing department, not its scientific department. In others, there is little evidence that the authors recruited for the report made substantial contribution to the research itself....Some of the authors listed in the Merck study reports of concern...question the true nature of ghostwriting. One neurologist originally listed as "External author and then listed as Dr. Leon J. Thal, of the University of California, San Diego in the final draft, died a year ago in an airplane crash.

An editorial by Drs. Psaty and Kronmal, published in the *Journal of the American Medical Association* (JAMA) that same year, also questioned whether Merck might have deliberately manipulated dozens of academic documents published in medical literature, in order to promote Vioxx under false pretenses.[46] The 1999 Vioxx study published in *JAMA* was not just flawed, it was most likely fraudulent.

Today in 2015, BioMed Central—an open access publisher of peer reviewed articles—is working with the international Committee on Publication Ethics (COPE) to tackle the broader problem of "perverse" incentives that reward scientists for "impact" and "productivity" rather than the quality of their research or the ability to replicate studies.

SEDUCING YOUR DOCTOR

The problem for you, the patient, is that you can't expect even the most well-meaning doctor to protect you from drugs like Vioxx and Celebrex, because the medical literature they rely on is at best biased and at worst dishonest. This is one reason why I rarely prescribe new drugs to my patients. I am painfully aware that Big Pharma is in it for the money, not your wellbeing. And historically too many of the "blockbuster" drugs turn out to be dangerous and unsafe. Think about it: Merck may have paid out a few hundred million in settlements over Vioxx, but that pales in comparison with the billions they made while the drug was on the market.

As a young physician in the 1990s, I first became aware of how deeply intertwined the practice of medicine is with pharmaceutical companies. It's like a grand seduction. It begins with the attractive and charming reps who come to the physicians' offices to lure him/her into creating "brand loyalty" to the particular drug they represent. Sad to say, most doctors are easy prey. We believe the studies drug reps show us are honest and truly represent the superiority of their drug. Keeping up with the newest drugs and scientific data is difficult when a doctor spends fifteen hours a day seeing 35-50 patients. The decision to treat with one drug versus another is a lot more arbitrary than you would think. Doctors rely on their pharmaceutical reps to help make these decisions.

By the end of the 1990s, I had decided to stop allowing drug reps into my office. Their presence and perfect pitches confused me. I was skeptical of their promises that "newer is always better," and that every new drug was a "breakthrough" and "safe" even if the FDA had approved it. As the Vioxx/Celebrex tragedy should remind us, FDA approval doesn't guarantee safety or efficacy. It became clear to me that I was more comfortable prescribing older drugs, with long track records used by millions of people over decades. I wasn't working in the ER, oncology or OR where life and death situations rely on the help of the newest drugs. Where I work we didn't need the newest blood pressure, arthritis, pain killer or sleeping pill. The proven ones with the longest track record were invariably the safest.

AN INSIDE JOB

When Dr. John Abramson discovered that the Vioxx and Celebrex studies published in highly respected medical journals had left vital information and warnings out of their reports, he learned this information from the FDA's own website. The FDA is charged with protecting us, the public, from dangerous drugs that can hurt us. So, if the FDA was aware of the dangers that were loud and clear in the data coming from Vioxx and Celebrex's early studies, why didn't they stop the publication of misleading articles? When asked this question, the FDA's response was that they, "could not constrain communication in a scientific journal," and that "this was a first amendment right of commercial speech issue." [47]

This is the same argument Big Pharma uses as their right to say whatever they want about their latest drug in a direct-to-consumer ad. I don't think this is a coincidence. Big Pharma and the FDA are pretty cozy partners. You see, the process of obtaining FDA approval and getting drugs out to the public is incredibly lengthy, complicated, and outrageously costly—to the tune of tens of millions of dollars. Only Big Pharma has the resources to get through such a process, which requires truckloads of data and multiple levels of trials—starting with animals and finishing up with humans—to prove a particular drug is safe and effective for a specific condition or disease. As you saw with the Merck example, once a drug gets FDA approval, the push begins to promote the drug and get as many prescriptions written as quickly as possible. To pharmaceutical companies, time is the enemy for a couple of reasons. First is the patent issue. Patent exclusivity is only good for a set amount of years.[48] Big profits are only made during that limited window the drug company owns the patent. Of significant note is the little known fact that the FDA only approves drugs for acute use for a six-week time periods so pharmaceutical companies don't technically have to prove long-term safety in their clinical data to get a drug approved. Thus, it becomes a race against time to sell as much as possible before potentially finding serious side effects and/or losing patent protection. Ironically, the FDA leaves the reporting of adverse effects up to the drug companies themselves. Self-reporting is dangerous and lends itself to many dishonorable practices.

The clock begins ticking the minute the FDA grants approval—or rather, when pharmaceutical corporations get the inside tip that they're going to get approval. That is when you'll start seeing those beautifully produced ads in mainstream, women's, and men's magazines, and on the Internet. Then radio and TV ad campaigns begin and hundreds of millions of dollars are spent by the pharmaceutical company, especially if the new drug is considered a potential "blockbuster." Books start appearing on the disease the new drug treats. Suddenly the need for the drug is everywhere you turn. At the same time the army of beautiful, charming young sales reps head out to charm the doctors who will prescribe the drug.

In 1998, when Pfizer brought Viagra to the market, the media was flooded with reports of the wonders of the drug. It was leading the way to a new sexual revolution! This little blue pill was the answer to every man's woes—and, apparently, every woman's—as those commercials with the smiling grey-haired couples so successfully proved. Within a few short months, men were inundating their doctors' offices, begging them to prescribe the drug. If they didn't want to lose their patients, doctors started writing scripts for Viagra.

Within a few short years, it became clear that the men who needed it the most couldn't really use it safely. The majority of "erectile dysfunction" cases—a disease made for television and insurance reimbursement—are caused by aging, cardiovascular problems, plaque deposition, atherosclerosis, obesity, diabetes, and lifestyle. In short: old age. But older men with heart disease, blood pressure problems, and vascular disease can't safely take Viagra. The drug causes a significant drop in blood pressure and even heart attacks. Pfizer has billions of dollars at stake in Viagra—they want the sales of the drug to last far longer than their customers' erections! So word on the street begins promoting Viagra as a drug for young men—to see how strong an erection they can have and how long they can last. Was Pfizer behind this new off label use for the drug? We'll never know. It's against the law for drug companies to suggest off-label use for their products, so we must give them the benefit of the doubt. But the end result is the same—Viagra continues to be a blockbuster drug and doctors prescribe it every day. In my practice I've prescribed it for young and old because, at the end of the day, men believe Viagra will save their libido.

SPEAK NO EVIL

Sadly, since drug companies are in charge of reporting the negative side effects of their own drugs to the FDA, reports of potentially dangerous side effects rarely see the light of day. That leaves the public and the medical profession in dangerous territory. Proving connections between drugs and certain side-effects is often difficult, but when drug companies slam the door in your face and don't even want to hear about it, it's impossible to help the patient or address the truth.

Cathy was a beautiful, effervescent twenty-four-year old woman I took care of for more than a decade in my internal medicine practice. I'd known her since she was a teenager; both she and her mother were my patients. When Cathy developed a mass in her breast, which a biopsy proved cancerous, we were all devastated. There was no medical history, no family history, no genetic or environmental connection. In fact, there was no reason for this young woman to have breast cancer. She was an athlete, ate an almost perfect diet, didn't drink, smoke, or take drugs. The mystery kept me up at night. Finally, I made a connection. For six years, since she was eighteen years old, I had been prescribing birth control pills for her.

At the time, there wasn't much published data linking birth control pills to cancer, but I started to wonder about a possible connection. Common sense told me that since birth control pills suppress a woman's hormone production down to menopausal levels and the risk of breast cancer increases after menopause, perhaps it was the pill that caused the cancer. It may not have been based on "evidence based" scientific research, but I was convinced there was a logical connection worth pursuing and after all the "evidence" was Cathy. Because I cared about my patient and my profession I thought it only right to try to find out if anyone else had made a similar connection. I called the pharmaceutical company that manufactured the pill she was taking and asked if they had any other reports of breast cancer in young women on that pill. My experience with this drug company was odd, to say the least. All I was trying to do was get information and report a possible side effect to the company that made, promoted, and sold birth control pills to the tune of millions of dollars a day. Instead of getting help, I got the runaround. I was referred through at least five layers of the company. It took me a week to get to the medical director in charge of the birth control pill division. From the moment I started asking him about any reports of possible connections between birth control pills and breast cancer, he tried to get me off the phone and bluntly told me there was no connection. He told me I had no way to prove any connection and hung up. As a consequence of that conversation, I started to believe there was a connection and still do to this day. Today, that connection is being made by many physicians around the country and research and books are proving us right.

I took Cathy off birth control pills and she had a short course of chemo. The tumor disappeared, never to return. I never prescribed birth control pills again.

MY EXPERIENCE WITH "LITTLE PHARMA"

In 2002, in the wake of the Women's Health Initiative—the failed NIH study on Premarin and Prempro, drugs used to treat menopausal symptoms of hot flashes and vaginal atrophy—I started my own compounding pharmacy (a pharmacy that created individualized preparations of hormones specific for the individual patient use), in my office in a suburb of New York City. One of my patient's husbands, a very successful medical advertising executive, became my partner in the pharmacy and promised to help grow the pharmacy with me. What he did was astounding. Within a few months, he had created beautiful marketing materials, made the pharmacy a presence at trade shows, sent me on the road to give lectures to doctors at dinners the pharmacy sponsored—a regular press junket. It was a huge eye opener for me— the first time I actually saw firsthand pharmaceutical marketing. Sadly, the business end of the pharmacy couldn't survive the enormous strain of the massive spending my partner undertook to promote it. Since we weren't a large drug company or a manufacturer with unlimited funds and since my interest lay more in educating doctors and treating patients than in promoting bioidentical hormone preparations—we decided to part ways even though the business was growing rapidly, with more than a hundred doctors prescribing to the pharmacy within less than one year.

I was actually relieved to get out of the business end of medicine anyway. My goal has always been to be a good doctor, to care for my patients, and to share my experience with other doctors. Eventually my partner returned to his lucrative marketing career in Big Pharma. He raved about how much money there was to be made working for Big Pharma, creating advertising for drugs. He'd smirk and say that doctors came cheap. A free dinner at a fancy restaurant is all it takes to buy their loyalty. The experience saddened me. How many doctors are aware they are being used as unpaid sales people for Big Pharma?

My initial reaction was to turn against drug companies altogether and focus on teaching patients to stay away from medications. I was disappointed and had lost faith in Big Pharma. But in time I realized that was an extreme reaction. When properly researched, prescribed, and taken correctly, pharmaceuticals will improve and save many lives. With more experience I realized the best way I could help my patients was to integrate the use of prescription medication with supplements, bio-identical hormones, diet, exercise, lifestyle, sleep, and stress management. That's when I realized the best way to practice good medicine after listening to the patient, is to provide support from both conventional and integrative standpoints.

Unfortunately, I am only one of a handful of doctors who see things so broadly. Doctors typically stay on either the conventional or the alternative side of the discussion. The inability to meet in the middle and make use of the best of both sides for the good of the patient is a sad commentary on my profession.

I could go on forever with examples of how Big Pharma has taken over our entire healthcare system and capitalized—both overtly and covertly—on our fears of dying or missing a deadly disease. Every day new books and papers prove that pharmaceutical companies are leading us in a dangerous direction.

Boniva for "osteopenia", low bone density that is less severe than osteoporosis (another made-for-TV disease); Adderall for ADD, and a staple drug for millions of college students with "trouble concentrating"; Zoloft and Lexapro antidepressants used for hot flashes; Nexium for heartburn and acid reflux; a never-ending procession of painkillers; sleeping pills galore. The list goes on and on. We have become a nation addicted to prescription medications. There are thousands more examples of how Big Pharma creates diseases and your doctor writes the prescription for their drugs. The false sense of security you get from the FDA and prestigious medical journals is just part of the tragedy. The truth is, when it comes to taking medications—prescription or over-the-counter—you are out there on your own. That may sound scary if you want to be the "perfect patient," but to me it is a blessing in disguise. Understanding the situation may force you to begin to make your own medical decisions without putting undue trust onto the doctor, insurance, or drug company. Take your time, honestly evaluate your lifestyle, and make the necessary changes, and only as a last resort consider the drugs.

CHAPTER 6
HOSPITALS WILL MAKE YOU SICK

"I am dying from the treatment of too many physicians."
—Alexander The Great

Having worked in hospitals for more than two decades, including serving as medical director of the emergency room of a large academic trauma center in the suburbs of New York City, I can tell you unequivocally that *unless you are in mortal danger the best thing you can do is stay away from hospitals.*

If you are acutely ill—if you are in a motor vehicle accident, have a heart attack, have acute exacerbations of chronic diseases like obstructive pulmonary disease or liver failure, if you can't breathe without assistance, or are bleeding uncontrollably—you certainly *need* hospital care.

According to a 2013 American Hospital Association survey there are 5,724 hospitals in the U.S.: 2,903 are nonprofit, 1,025 are for profit and 1,045 are owned by state or local government entities.

Academic medical centers are hospitals that are affiliated with medical schools. They have accredited training programs for medical students, interns, residents, and fellows and they also conduct clinical research along with patient care. They are designated as tertiary care centers because they offer a full range of treatments from major trauma care in their emergency rooms, to transplants, open heart surgery, and a wide array of subspecialists. There are around four hundred of these centers in the U.S. Examples include: New York-Presbyterian, Bellevue/ NYU, Kings County Hospital/Downstate, Johns Hopkins/Baltimore City, Jacobi/ Einstein, Mayo Clinic, Cleveland Clinic, Cornell Weil, University of Pittsburgh Medical Center Presbyterian.

About 53% of hospitals in the U.S. are part of a health system. The number is constantly growing, changing the landscape of hospital ownership and turning them into major businesses. According to Irving Levin in 2012 these business transactions amounted to $1.88 billion and represented ninety-four mergers and acquisitions.

The largest for profit hospital operators are: Hospital Corporation of America (162 hospitals), Community Health Systems (135 hospitals), and Health Management Associates (71 hospitals).

The largest not-for-profit hospitals in the U.S. by number of beds are: New York Presbyterian Hospital (New York City) >2200 beds, Florida Hospital Orlando >2100 beds, and Jackson Memorial Hospital Miami >1700 beds.

In-patient hospital admissions are on the decline due to a general shift to outpatient care driven primarily by advances in minimally invasive surgeries that don't require overnight stays and anesthesia techniques that allow for faster patient recovery after surgical procedures.

Hospital care is confusing and often of poor quality because of the way the system works. No one is at the helm of individual patient care and thus no one takes full responsibility for the outcome. This leads to too many tests, too many subspecialists, too many surgeries and medications, and confusing information, all dangerous for the patient and horrifying for the families. Imagine an airplane without a pilot— how would you like to be one of the passengers on it?

My patient, and contributor to this book, Victoria Reggio, shares her own family's all too common tragic experience with this disorganized system:

GOOD RIDDANCE, ST. JOHN'S

As a lifelong New Yorker, I am usually saddened when I learn of a hospital shutting down, but I breathed a sigh of relief when I learned that St. John's in Elmhurst, Queens was closing its doors.

On a Saturday in April, 2008, my brother, Ron, called from my mother's apartment telling me he was taking her to St. John's emergency room for a badly infected toe and leg. She was eighty-seven years old, the infection was diabetes-related, and her podiatrist was affiliated with St. John's.

After several hours, Ron called from the emergency room.

"Vicki, we've been here for hours and no one has seen her. Mom is really in pain. I don't know what to do." I could tell by the sound of his voice, he was panicking.

"Ron, did they ask about her history, take her temperature?"

"They haven't done a damn thing. She's sitting here with a slipper on her foot because we couldn't put a sneaker on it; it's that swollen. I have to go. Let me see if I can get a doctor to look at her."

By early evening, several guards made their rounds and told my brother to leave. Ron left hoping mom was going to be taken to a room shortly.

The next morning, I joined Ron and we went to the hospital. We were horrified to find mom still in the emergency room. She was lying on a gurney in a great deal of pain.

I approached the desk and begged for someone to give my mother some attention. The nurse barely looked at me and said, "She'll be given something shortly." Four hours later and twenty-four hours after she arrived at the emergency room, my mother received some pain medication, food, something to drink, and help with a bedpan. A technician drew her blood.

It was now close to her second evening at the hospital and she still didn't have a room. Once again, surly guards came around and my brother and I were ordered to leave. Leaving my defenseless mother in the care of such incompetents was unsettling, but as we weighed our options and spoke to a nurse we were assured my mom would be moved to a room soon and would be better off in the hospital than in her own apartment.

I was awakened at 6:00 a.m. by a phone call from Ron.

"Vicki, the hospital called. Mom fell and they want us there as soon as possible."

We went there in a frenzy. We were directed to her room. It was filthy, smelled horrible and my mother was not there. Scared out of my mind I went to the nursing station where the head nurse told me that my mother was having a scan on another floor. We found her just as they were wheeling her out of the radiology suite. A doctor said that she fell during the night, shortly after she was brought to her room.

I was enraged and screamed at the doctor.

"How the hell could my mother fall out of bed when she can't even turn without pain? How could this happen?" The doctor was clearly shaken but politely continued saying that after she fell out of the bed she suffered a heart attack. This was like a bad dream. There was no explanation why she fell, nor why she had a heart attack.

My mother was brought to the cardiac care unit, where her treatment was marginally better. The nurses were attentive, but the doctors were arrogant and rude. My mother was restrained—arms and legs tied to the bed rails—supposedly to prevent her from falling and at one point, a doctor came into her cubicle, did a perfunctory examination, ignored us and left without a word.

I ran after him and in front of the nurses shouted, "Stop. What's your name?"

"I'm Dr. M."

"Well, Dr. M you just ignored my brother and me when you examined my mother. How dare you not even acknowledge our presence? She's in this situation because she fell in this horrible hospital. What is wrong with you?"

My brother came running out to calm me down.

I apologized and asked the doctor to please introduce himself and explain what was going on with my mother. He just kept walking away ignoring us. There are no words to describe how I felt at this point.

Another doctor announced that they were going to do another (unnamed) test, requiring an injection. By this time, we had contacted my mother's cardiologist, who said he would call the hospital and speak to one of the doctors. Up to that point not one single doctor or nurse had asked about her medical history. Once the cardiologist gave the hospital my mother's history, she was promptly transferred to Long Island Jewish Hospital in the care of her cardiologist.

When my mother arrived at LIJ, we learned that she had indeed suffered a massive heart attack after the fall. Her face was bruised from the fall and the (unnamed) scan requiring the injection done at St. John's had caused liver damage (from the dye).

Somehow, my mother survived her ordeal at St. John's. She was at LIJ for many weeks and was discharged to a nursing home where she stayed until she passed on November 13, 2008. She had gone from living in her own apartment independently to becoming a statistic in our broken healthcare system.

The media portrayed the closing of St. John's as a tragedy. In reality, this hospital had a horrible reputation, particularly when it came to emergency services. It did not serve the community and quite frankly, a hospital like this is more dangerous than no hospital at all.

GET OUT WHILE YOU CAN

Often patients will complain that they, or a loved one, were discharged from the hospital too soon. Their reasoning seems logical: wouldn't it have been better to have good quality supervised care, rather than being pushed out before feeling better? The answer is not always *yes*. In fact, too often it is a resounding *NO*.

Hospitals are among the worst places to be if you're sick. In fact, our own federal government's Department of Health and Human Services—Office of Inspector General conducts ongoing research to identify severity of the dangers and investigates methods to improve the reporting of adverse effects in hospitalized patients. [49]

Hospital mistakes account for around $33 billion in preventable costs and kill more than 31,000 patients a year. The Institute of Medicine estimates that as many as 100,000 Americans die each year from preventable medical errors in hospitals,[50] This is nearly triple the roughly 34,000 people who are killed every year in automobile accidents. Two hundred 747 airplanes would have to crash, killing everyone on board, to equal the number of people who die from "reported" medical errors in hospitals. Experts have said that medical mistakes are the third-leading cause of death in the United States. That makes hospitals an extremely dangerous place indeed.

Hospitals are most dangerous for the elderly. Although we are constantly told that life expectancy has improved over the past five decades, too many older Americans suffer with multiple chronic ailments, such as arthritis, diabetes, COPD, high blood pressure, and dementia (Alzheimer's). In an interview by Jonathan Rauch of *Atlantic Magazine*, Joanne Lynn, the director of the Altarum Institute Center for Elder Care and Advanced Illness stated, "A gradual and medically complicated downslide was once exceptional...but is now the likely path for half of today's elders." [51] The problem is that every time an elderly person enters a hospital their health declines exponentially faster than if they had stayed home.[52] For many, just one hospitalization results in a downturn in health and quality of life that may well be irreversible. A recent study showed that out of sixty well-functioning, independent adults seventy-five years or older who were admitted to the hospital from their home for acute illness, a staggering 75 percent were no longer able to live independently after release, including 15 percent who were discharged directly to nursing homes.[53] This study found that the main source of this decline wasn't the progression of the illness they'd been admitted for, but rather complications associated with the hospital stay, including unnecessary and lengthy bed rest (bedsores, muscle atrophy, weakness), urinary tract infections, pneumonia, and psychological stressors caused by taking a person out of their home and placing them in an unfamiliar environment—all of which are particularly detrimental and deadly to elderly patients. (Vicki's mother's story is sadly the perfect example.)

THE GERM FACTORY

Ignaz Semmelweiss, a physician in Vienna, Austria, during the 1840s became concerned with the high numbers of women dying of puerperal (a.k.a. childbed fever), bacterial infections following childbirth. He noted that women giving birth with midwives had a much lower incidence of puerperal fever, compared to those giving birth with the help of doctors in the hospital's maternity ward. He made the connection that many of the medical students who cared for the women had performed autopsies just prior to visiting and helping with labor and delivery.

Once he made this connection, Semmelweiss instituted a requirement for all doctors to wash their hands with chlorinated lime before assisting with deliveries. The result was a dramatic decrease in the number of deaths on Dr. Semmelweiss's ward. Unfortunately, it was many years before the medical establishment adopted this visionary's commonsense practice.

Semmelweiss was fired from his job, and died in a mental institution at the age of forty-seven. The doctors in his hospital were furious at the implication that it was *their* fault women were dying and refused to take responsibility. Sadly, it is human nature to refuse to accept novel ideas that question the status quo. While thinking out of the box is encouraged and rewarded in other professions, medicine is notoriously backward in its approach to innovations in patient care. Unfortunately, this reticence to growth and change in medicine may cost lives.[54]

Refusing to consider new ideas is, tragically, typical of academic medicine. Because of this situation, most advances in medicine come from the private sector, where innovation is welcomed, encouraged, and rewarded. Academic medicine is too much about politics, manipulation, and negative reinforcement. Skepticism is the rule and listening is not an option.

Today, everybody knows the relationship between germs and infections; between washing your hands and preventing germs from spreading. Despite this knowledge in our modern world, just like in the 1800s, hospitals are still breeding grounds for deadly infections. An estimated two-and-a-half million patients develop *nosocomial* (hospital-acquired) infections while in the hospital. These infections are resistant to antibiotics, making them deadlier than ever. In many ways, the landscape of infectious diseases is a lot more dangerous today than it was in the 1800s.

Compounding the problem is the way hospital administrators and physicians cover up the facts. Hospitals are actively keeping you, the patient, from finding out their true infection rates. And, in many places around the country, the government is turning a blind eye to the problem.

In researching the back story of a case in Los Angeles, in which a cardiac surgeon unknowingly spread a staph infection from his hands to the hearts of as many as sixty patients on whom he operated, *LA Times* investigative journalist Melody Petersen[55] uncovered a strict policy of silence among federal, state, and local health investigators across the country. Public health officials defend this deadly code of silence, stating hospitals are trustworthy and will self-regulate. What they're really doing is putting the fox in charge of the chicken coop. Self-reporting is a dangerous practice that is used in multiple areas of the healthcare industry (remember pharmaceutical companies self-report on side effects of their drugs), with deadly outcomes. In places like Los Angeles County, even when hospitals are found to have high incidences of reportable infections, they don't face any fines or penalties; business continues as usual, at the expense of thousands of patients who fall victim to hospital-acquired infections.

And, without being aware of potentially life-saving information, other hospitals don't correct problems that could save countless lives. In the second article of her investigation, Petersen gives the example of a case in Florida in late 2008, where the use of one simple piece of faulty medical equipment—a hard-to-sterilize duodenoscope (part of an endoscope)—spread the deadly intestinal bacteria and "superbug" CRE, which is lethal in up to 50 percent of those infected. After fifteen patients died, the hospital reported the incident to the CDC (Centers for Disease Control) and the FDA—and that's where the story ends. No one else in the medical community heard of it again, until four years later, when the Florida case was written up in a professional medical journal by the doctors involved. By then, investigators had connected the use of the *very same defective piece of equipment* to more CRE outbreaks—and hundreds more preventable deaths had occurred in several other states. To this day the CDC and state authorities still defend the clearly failed "self-reporting" model of dealing with hospital infections.

THE LATEST IN DEADLY INFECTIONS

One of the most dangerous bacteria to have reared its ugly head is called carbapenem-resistant Enterobacteriaceae or CRE. This bacteria is antibiotic-resistant and kills up to 50 percent of those infected. The CDC has called the bacteria "a family of nightmare superbugs." Some CRE bacteria are resistant to almost all existing antibiotics. CRE is most dangerous to sick people (those likely to be found in hospitals); who are immunologically deficient, have chronic illnesses, are ventilator-dependent, and/or have urinary or intravenous catheters.

The CDC recommends that patients who are in hospitals or long-term care facilities, insist their healthcare professionals wash their hands before touching them, clean their own hands often, inform their doctors if they've recently been hospitalized in another facility, and not overdo the use of antibiotics. But then, how many people read CDC recommendations, or even know they exist? **It's unconscionable that enforcing CDC recommendations is made the patient's responsibility, not the responsibility of the hospital and every employee working there.**

Think about all the people who work and spend time in training hospitals who come into direct contact with patients: doctors, interns, residents, nurses, nursing assistants, attendants, technicians, dieticians, therapists, housekeeping staff, administrative staff, aides, friends, and family. Do all these people wash their hands before coming into contact with each patient? Not likely.

THE TRUTH ABOUT HAND SANITIZERS

What about those hand sanitizer dispensers installed outside elevators or rooms in your highly-rated hospital? Don't they protect you? Here's some unsettling news about those dispensers and the bottle you keep by your bedside: alcohol-based hand sanitizers aren't anywhere near as effective as you've been led to believe.[56] In 2005, a group of Boston doctors published the first in-home clinical trials on the efficacy of alcohol-based hand sanitizers. They enrolled three hundred local families with young children in daycare and instructed them to use hand sanitizers aggressively. Researchers found the incidence of respiratory infections among the children who used the sanitizers did not change from those who did not use them. In New York, a Columbia University study based on inner-city families produced similar results, as did an epidemiologic study by Allison Aiello at the University of Michigan. Three years later, in 2008, the Boston study was repeated, with the same results. While Purell may kill viruses in controlled, laboratory conditions, it's not nearly as reliable in the real world. Today, 169 years after Semmelweiss' simple solution, a thorough hand washing with soap and hot water remains our best guarantee for preventing the transmission of germs.

Unfortunately, risk of infection is only one part of the story. Even world-renowned hospitals, with low infection rates, can treat patients in such a neglectful, impersonal, and piecemeal manner that they risk not only the spread of infection, but also the creation of more problems and complications. The following story is even more distressing because it happened to a world-renowned surgeon. Many doctors are treated like VIPs in their own hospitals, but this doctor had to go to another facility to have the back surgery she needed. There she experienced the whole process through the eyes of a normal, regular patient. If a medically savvy person like this surgeon can't get decent hospital care, then what hope is there for the average human being? The following story is told in the doctor's own words:

DR. R'S STORY

I had a two-level (L3-L4-L5) lumbar (spinal) fusion performed at a world-renowned New York hospital on Wednesday, December 19, 2012. After the surgery, I think my surgeon told me that everything was great—although, at the time I was in the recovery room, still drowsy from anesthesia. That day, I was on an on-demand morphine pump for pain.

Thursday, my first full postoperative day, my doctor came by early in the morning for a visit. He looked at my back and told me that all was well. He asked if I had passed gas. I told him, maybe. But by noon I was aware that my GI (gastrointestinal) tract had completely shut down. I tried eating some cereal, but I could not swallow; stomach acid came into my mouth, and my abdomen (belly) began to swell.

That first day, no one listened to my lungs (or abdomen) and I never saw a respiratory therapist. As a surgeon, I know that patients often develop problems with their lungs after general anesthesia. A nurse eventually brought me an incentive spirometer (a device given to patients after surgery to help improve respiratory function) to help expand my lungs. I never saw a physical therapist or a resident that day. The pain management team came in for a thirty-second visit and switched me to oral pain medications. Surprisingly, no one asked me about my prior experience with pain medication. I was placed on Percocet (two every six hours) with morphine shots and a muscle relaxant (Flexeril).

As the day wore on, my GI tract problem worsened to the point that my abdomen was so distended that I looked pregnant. I showed my nurse who reassured me that things would be okay soon. Throughout my entire hospital stay no one examined my abdomen. Every doctor and nurse who came to see me asked, "Passed gas?" like it was a rhetorical question. I knew that my GI system was blocked and nothing was moving through. It is a very common side-effect of narcotic painkillers.

Despite my inability to eat, regular meals continued to be brought to my bedside. In fact, the only people who made reliable visits to me were from the dietary department. I also had a low-grade fever and symptoms of a urinary tract infection, including burning on urination, frequency, and urgency. A medical consultation was requested and I gave a urine sample for the lab to analyze.

That evening at about 10 p.m., I was suddenly taken to the X-ray department for X-rays of my back. No one told me why. A wheelchair without back support was brought in. I thought to myself, "Has no one ever considered a better or safer way to transport a fresh back-surgery patient?" I tried to get in the ridiculous chair, and then announced, "I am not going anywhere in this." Eventually, an old-fashioned, over-sized wheelchair appeared. The X-ray was done quickly, and I asked for the results. Was everything all right? The technician didn't know. A few hours later, I asked the nurse to find out if my back X-rays were okay. "They're not in the system yet," she said. Over the following two days, I was given the same answer many times. Even to the day of my discharge, I was still unable to get anyone to tell me if the results of my X-rays were okay. Like all patients, I was thinking that something must be wrong. It would have been nice for someone to communicate with me, to let me know what was going on.

Now comes the really scary part. Later that evening, I was still in pain but afraid to sleep. I was especially concerned about taking Flexeril in combination with high doses of narcotics. Indeed, half a Flexeril put me to sleep immediately. I demanded to have a pulse oximeter (an oxygen monitor) and hired a private duty nurse to watch me at night and wake me if I stopped breathing. People die in hospitals because they stop breathing. Unfortunately, this happens fairly commonly.[57] It's called "respiratory arrest," and guess what usually causes that? Too high dosing of narcotic painkillers like the ones I was given. I believe that had I taken all the medication as prescribed by the pain management team, I might have died.

On Friday, post-operative day two, my surgeon came in early, but I was too overmedicated to have a meaningful conversation. Anything I ate came right back up. No one seemed concerned.

That afternoon, I finally got my wish to see a physical therapist. As I was walking down the hall, the therapist watched me from afar, and quickly gave me a smiling thumbs-up, "Walking. Good job. I'll sign you out." That, apparently, was my entire physical therapy consultation! Wait. What about my questions? What about walking, how much? Sitting? Best position for sleeping? Stretching? Rolling over? I had so many crucial questions that were never even addressed.

I was discharged three days after surgery, an hour after my surgical drains were removed. I was sent home without any homecare. No surgical wound care. No home-health nurse. No social worker. No physical therapist. No physician.

As I was on my way out the door on a Saturday, with a black car waiting, engine running, I put on the hospital-issued back-brace and one of the strings broke. Since it was almost Christmas, I wondered if I could get a replacement. Standing at the front desk, the unit secretary offered, "Let me call Jane, the orthopedic resident; they may have a bunch of them in a closet somewhere."

Not long thereafter, a young woman got off the elevator. When she passed me, I smiled and asked, "Hi, are you Jane, the orthopedic resident?" She did not even acknowledge me. She certainly heard me. I waited a couple of minutes, and then I returned to the nurse's station. The young woman, Jane, didn't look at me. It was apparent that she was trying not to engage me. Her body language clearly said, "I will get to you when, and if, I am ready." Finally, I interrupted, "Excuse me are you Jane, the orthopedic resident? Did you not see me? Did you not hear me? You walked right by me at the elevator?"

Glaring, she acknowledged she was Jane the orthopedic resident. She was clearly angry that I did not call her "Doctor" and it was also clear that she felt imposed upon by my behavior and sheer existence. I asked about my broken belt and she told me that she couldn't help. She then turned back to the nurse in a rude, completely dismissive manner and that was it. The orthopedic resident, was completely unconcerned about my welfare. Her haughtiness toward and disdain for me, a patient in need of assistance, was shocking.

Oh, and guess who actually signed me out of the hospital? Jane, the orthopedic resident! Ironically, she was the doctor who filled out my INDIVIDUALIZED PATIENT DISCHARGE PLAN and signed her name to it. The plan said, "Outpatient Treatment plan discussed with patient." That was a blatant lie. I never saw her or spoke to her until that very unpleasant confrontation as I was going out the door. Jane signed me out without ever seeing me or talking to me. Isn't that fraud, misconduct, and malpractice?

To put this entire horrendous experience in perspective, I am a surgeon. Under no circumstances would I ever take care of a patient the way I was treated. Had those people who were involved in my care worked for me in any capacity, they would all have been fired. This was not good medicine.

SECRETS OF THE ER

During the years I spent in emergency medicine, I was passionate about my work. It was highly stressful, the hours were long, and every day I felt the weight of responsibility for the lives under my care. More frequently than other doctors, ER physicians have the experience of actually relieving excruciating pain, dealing with natural and manmade disasters, and saving lives. Ironically, the clinical detachment that is indoctrinated into us in medical school actually comes in handy in an emergency room. You, the patient, *definitely* don't want your physician reacting emotionally to the sight of a mangled body, a cardiac arrest, or the bloody mess left in the wake of a car accident. You want your

ER physician to be calm and collected; to focus on one thing and one thing only—saving your life. That doesn't mean ER personnel, in general, should be remote and distant toward their patients; quite the opposite. When I ran the ER, I made sure the doctors who worked with me always treated patients with respect and kindness. Regardless of specialty, better patient outcomes are universal when the patients feel cared for—even in the ER. It's high time all physicians took this to heart and patients stopped making allowances for rude and uncaring doctors.

One thing I learned in the ER is how to tell the difference between a true emergency and a health scare that would best be handled by a visit to the family doctor or even commonsense care at home. Our grandparents didn't run to the ER every time something went wrong. Some of them had the luxury of a doctor who made house calls, but generally, they were taken care of by their families until they could get a medical opinion or got better on their own. Today, the ER has become a catch-all providing care to everyone from the critically injured, to a child with a bad case of poison ivy, to an overweight middle-aged man whose sciatica is acting up.

Abuse and overuse of the ER has led to overcrowding in emergency rooms around the country—yet another sign of our broken system. If more patients had a relationship with a family primary care physician, who knew their history and with whom they could communicate on the phone, via email or text before rushing to the ER, those patients who are truly critical would get the care they need and those who only need reassurance and rest would stay out of harm's way. To improve the system, patients must connect with their primary care doctors *before* going to the ER or urgicenter commonly known as urgent care centers. A visit to the ER should be a last resort, not a first knee-jerk reaction.

A CLOSE CALL

Hank is a ridiculously healthy, fifty-two-year-old actor, in great shape and determined to stay that way. When Hank was a strapping young man of thirty, a bacterial infection (endocarditis) from a sloppy dental procedure and a mildly damaged heart valve caused a rare infection in his heart that ate away at his aortic valve. Hank was fine until one day, while performing in a play out of state, he started to become weak, tired, and short of breath. He got very sick very quickly and almost died of heart failure. Fortunately, he had an excellent cardiac surgeon, who replaced his infected aortic valve with a titanium valve. The surgery was a great success and Hank remains healthy to this day, though he is on a blood thinner (Coumadin) which protects him from forming blood clots on his prosthetic valve. To make sure his blood stays thin, he must test his blood clotting factors monthly. He takes a blood test and reports the results to his cardiologist.

Fast-forward twenty-two years. During a busy morning at the gym, Hank was doing bench presses with very heavy weights when he felt a pain like an electric shock run through his head. He "browned out" for a moment and then felt incredibly nauseous and dizzy. For a moment, he thought he was having a stroke. The incident ended as quickly as it began. Still, Hank was shaken. He hurried home and told his wife, Judith, what happened. By now, the episode had passed completely, but they contacted their family doctor by email just in case. Their doctor phoned back immediately. He was happy to hear the episode had passed, but because of Hank's history and the Coumadin (the drug that thinned his blood and increased the risk of bleeding) he recommended Hank get a CT scan of his brain to rule out the possibility of even a minor brain bleed. The doctor offered to set up the CT scan appointment for the next morning, but Hank was nervous. Rather than wait he and his wife decided to go to the emergency room of the prominent academic center they lived near.

At the ER, Hank gave the admitting nurse in the waiting room his complete medical history—including stressing the heart valve replacement and the Coumadin he was taking daily—then gave the exact same information again to the physician's assistant who did another intake in the ER proper. A phlebotomist drew his blood, an aide wheeled him in for a CT scan, and a resident did a quick physical and a neurologic exam. After that, Hank and Judith were left alone. They waited nearly two hours, holding hands and quietly reading their Kindles. Finally, a new doctor arrived; a neurologist. He was older, tall, and imposing, unquestionably, the authority. He looked at Hank's EMR, his blood and CT scan results, examined him without saying a word, and then took the nurse aside and whispered something to her. He walked out before either Hank or Judith could even ask his name or what his thoughts or findings were.

"What's wrong? What's going on?" Judith asked the nurse.

"He's going to be moved to the neurology floor," said the nurse.

"Why?"

"You'll have to ask the doctor," the nurse said quietly, before she too left the room to disappear into the chaos of the bustling ER.

An orderly came into the small room and told Hank that he was taking him "upstairs." Hank was compliant, but Judith was getting angry. She stormed out of the room and managed to track down the first doctor they'd seen, the young resident who'd examined Hank when he first came into the ER. Judith demanded, in no uncertain terms, that they be told what was happening. Fortunately, the resident wasn't too busy so she stopped and actually listened to Judith, knitting her brow as she went to the nursing station and opened Hank's medical record. "Hmmm," she said. "Dr. T has ordered a spinal tap. He is the attending physician here. That means whatever he says gets done."

"WHAT?!! A spinal tap? Why?" Judith couldn't believe what she was hearing. She was a writer and didn't know much about medicine, but she knew that a spinal tap was an invasive procedure. Unless there was evidence of infection or some other serious neurologic problem she couldn't imagine

why the neurologist who had barely seen Hank would order such a drastic procedure. The resident obligingly looked through Hank's chart again and shook her head, "I don't know. CT scan's normal. Blood work is normal. Doesn't seem to have any sign of infection. Neurologic exam was normal. But Dr. T is the head of neurology so he must have a good reason."

This answer didn't satisfy Judith. Because of the blood-thinning effect of Coumadin, she knew Hank couldn't safely undergo elective surgery or procedure without specific preparations. He risked bleeding to death. She told this to the resident. "He's on Coumadin! He shouldn't have a spinal tap or any procedure unless it's a matter of life or death."

The resident raised her eyebrows, "Why didn't you let anyone know he was on Coumadin?"

Now Judith was really furious, not at the resident, who was clearly trying to be helpful, but at the entire situation. She struggled to keep her composure. "We told the nurse when we arrived, we told the PA as well, and my husband wears a giant med-alert tag stating he's on Coumadin!! It should be all over his record!"

*The resident took a second look at the EMR and sure enough, there it was in bold caps on the first page: **MEDICATIONS: COUMADIN**.*

"I'll get this information to Dr. T," she said, trying to sound casual. Meanwhile, Judith saw out of the corner of her eye that Hank was being wheeled out of his ER cubicle toward the elevator. She rushed back to Hank's side and told the orderly he would not be moved until she'd spoken with the doctor. There was a short silence but both Hank and Judith held their ground.

After about forty-five minutes of waiting, the resident returned with a new doctor in tow—he introduced himself as Dr. S, a fellow on the neurology service. He asked Hank a series of specific questions (beginning with asking him if he really was on Coumadin and, if so, why), then he read Hank's EMR all over again. He looked a little pale. "I think there's been some confusion," Dr. S said "It looks as if everything's normal, so we're going to discharge you." Judith and Hank were stunned. They tried to ask the newest member of the healthcare team for some explanation of what had happened, but were met with a wall of silence. Happy to have survived the nightmare, they hurried out of the crazy hospital.

In the taxi on the way home, Hank kissed Judith and held her close. "I don't know what would've happened to me if you hadn't been there," he said. "It all happened so fast, I never would have thought the old Coumadin would be a problem." By questioning the process, standing her ground, and requesting Hank get noticed and treated as an individual; Judith had clearly saved her husband from a potentially dangerous situation.

While Hank's decision to go to the ER is totally understandable, it points out the potential dangers associated with entering the system from a position of fear. The story as told by his wife inspires sympathy and compassion, but more importantly it should motivate us to take responsibility for protecting ourselves from a system we are brought up to trust, but which sadly is more likely to harm us.

CONSPIRACY OF SILENCE

Few humans know how to admit they are wrong and take ownership of their mistakes. Doctors, in particular, cannot afford to sweep mistakes under the carpet, yet very few have the courage to accept responsibility for their missteps. This problem is even more dangerous in hospitals, often run by administrators and doctors who don't own up to their mistakes. Because of this dangerous flaw, the healthcare profession often places patients in life-endangering situations. Competing for patients, in constant fear of lawsuits, both doctors and hospitals truly conspire to keep their mistakes behind closed doors. The secrecy surrounding deadly infections is just the tip of the iceberg when it comes to hospital errors. A sad wall of silence surrounds the unspoken agreement that doctors do not report other doctors who are impaired by alcohol, drugs, or other debilitating problems. Doctors within a clique always protect their colleagues. Hospitals will collude to hide a bad doctor's performance as long as s/he is a high volume producer; meaning, if the doctor makes money for the hospital, fills beds, performs many surgeries, the hospital and fellow doctors will do everything in their power to keep the doctor working, regardless of the danger he is to himself or the patients he cares for.

When I was a young doctor, I found myself in the middle of just such a hospital cover up:

Within a few short months of working with Dr. Jones, in my early thirties, I discovered that he had a terrible drug and alcohol problem. Soon after, I was very surprised to learn that most other physicians, as well as the administrators of the hospital at which he had been an attending for decades, were well aware of his addiction, yet not one doctor or nurse or administrator had reported him or—more importantly—offered to get him help. The hospital just wanted to keep him working because he had a huge practice and kept the hospital beds full. He was also a consistent source of revenue for the dozens of subspecialists who benefitted from his referrals. After a few months of working with him, seeing him treating patients while under the influence, I felt compelled to tell him that I would report him if he did not get treatment. He just ignored me. I went to the head of the medicine department at the hospital and tried, as compassionately as I could, to explain the problem and ask for help. The medical director, an elderly man himself, looked at me with total disdain. He told me, in no uncertain terms, that I had made a grave mistake by coming in to report the good doctor. He told me not to "stir the pot," to mind my own business, and to keep my mouth shut; warning me that talking about the doctor's problem would create far more problems for me than it would for Dr. Jones.

It took me months to decide to take the matter further. Working with him was stressful. I never knew what to expect from one day to the next. There were times I had to ask him to go home and I'd take over all the work because he was in such bad shape. I learned that he had been in rehab before, and that gave me some hope. So I talked to him and begged him to stop seeing patients until he'd gotten the help he so desperately needed. After many unsuccessful attempts to convince him, I threatened to leave the practice. By then, he was in terrible shape. He could barely get out of bed and was missing most of his office hours. Finally, he gave me permission to report him, and together we found him an excellent rehab center that focused on physicians with addictions like his.

Once he left the practice and was admitted to the rehab center, things started to deteriorate for me at the hospital. As the chief of medicine had warned me, I became a pariah among my peers; labeled a "bad guy" for turning in a colleague. No one was thinking about the patients he may have harmed, or the poor doctor's desperate cry for help. My colleagues focused only on my violation of their code of silence.

As for Dr. Jones, his license to practice medicine was suspended by the state. When he came out of rehab, it was reinstated with certain limitations and he began to rebuild his life by working with other physicians with addiction problems. He found his new career to be his true calling, and developed a new passion for life. He became a star in the field, helping hundreds of doctors beat the habit, and ended his career with a great group of friends and a loyal following of doctors who would never have gotten the help they needed had it not been for Dr. Jones. Years later, he thanked me for saving his life. Just think, if I had been intimidated into joining into the code of silence, he probably wouldn't have survived, he very likely would have harmed countless patients, and he never would have had a second chance helping so many other doctors in desperate need of help.

Doctors are only human. Covering up for someone with an impairment that affects his/her performance as a physician only serves to perpetuate bad medical practice and reinforces the sense of arrogance and superiority so pervasive in my profession. Yet this happens so frequently in hospitals, it's frightening—and hospitals almost always keep their scandals under wraps.[58] As medical consumers, we need to demand transparency and a higher level of care from our doctors and hospitals. Without transparency and accountability, we will never have a hospital system we can or should trust.

KISSING ROUNDS—A BETTER WAY TO PRACTICE

In the mid-1980s after my experience with Dr. Jones, I went into private practice with another physician, Dr. Mario Dolan, in Irvington, New York, a middle class suburb of New York City. We had a thriving practice where the patients loved us and we loved them.

In Chapter 3, I explained the rise of the insurance companies as they monopolized medicine in the '80s. Despite the fact that malpractice and insurance changes were descending upon us, Dr. Dolan and I decided to fight the trend and continue practicing the type of medicine he believed in. Dr. Dolan called a defining part of his style of practice "kissing rounds." I was very young and academically oriented so I didn't much appreciate his old school approach to medical care. Today, with more than thirty-five years of practice under my belt, I have come to totally agree with his philosophy and practice. "Kissing rounds" were Sunday morning rounds Dr. D made in the hospital. He would sit on the patient's bed surrounded by the patient's family. It was a sight to behold.

As a clinician, Dr. D was not very up to date with the latest drugs or medical procedures available in academic centers, but the patients loved him and they did well under his care. I now believe that this was largely due to the fact that his patients knew he cared enough to give up his Sunday mornings to spend time with them when they were sick enough to be in the hospital. It took me about twenty years of following the pre-programmed, purely evidence-based clinical approach to medicine, before I came to understand that what he did in his "kissing rounds" sent patients home faster and healthier than many of the state-of-the-art and cutting-edge procedures and treatments to which I had been subjecting my patients in the quest for the highest quality medicine.

In time, I combined his way of practicing medicine with the one I had been trained in and we came up with a much more successful formula. Patients did not need to stay in the hospital or be subjected to an infinite number of tests with the sole purpose of finding something wrong. The relationship between patient and doctor was the most important part of our practice, supported by up-to-date, evidence-based medicine. It was a win-win for both of us and, most importantly, for our patients.

DOING HOSPITALS RIGHT

I don't want to leave you with the depressing thought that all hospitals give bad care and that there is no hope for a better future. There are indeed amazing hospitals out there, and there is excellent medical care available in the U.S. today. You've got to look for it— and demand it—but it's definitely there. Most good care is focused on making hospitals less daunting and scary and focusing on customer service, treating patients like people, not like numbers on an electronic chart. Some hospitals are turning to the hospitality industry for inspiration and much needed advice on how to better transform their institutions into places where patients will feel less frightened and helpless—in short, making them less *institutional*. Providing more private and semi-private rooms; updating their environment with clean, bright, and freshly painted walls, artwork and furniture that remind of a comfortable hotel rather than a hospital; improving menus so that meals are fresher, healthier and tastier; encouraging open visiting hours so that patients are never without the support of their families and friends; and creating an atmosphere of empathy and kindness, designed to relieve stress rather than augment it—these are some of the ways healthcare pioneers and mavericks are working to improve hospital care.

Two areas of medicine that are making positive strides and leading the way in improved, cutting-edge care are the specialties of plastic surgery (elective procedure) and maternity medicine. Our family had a most remarkable experience with the latter.

In the fall of 2014, my daughter delivered my grand-twins at Mt. Sinai Hospital in Miami, Florida. The care she received was superb. Her obstetrician, Dr. Maurizio Bitran, a Chilean-trained physician who has been in practice in Miami for more than two decades, was caring, compassionate, and devoted; an outstanding clinician and human being. If all physicians were like Dr. Maurizio Bitran and the maternity staff at Mt. Sinai, our healthcare system would indeed be the best in the world.

From the moment our family set foot in the hospital the night before the twins were expected, caring, responsive and kind nurses, aides, technicians, clerical and administrative personnel and assistants all embraced my daughter and son-in-law with a well-coordinated expression of support. We immediately felt like welcome guests and not for a moment did we feel the care was less than personal and individualized. The labor rooms were pristine, up to date, and tastefully decorated in peaceful and cheery colors. Hospital services rivaled a hotel's amenities. The meals were not just edible, they were delicious and beautifully presented. During the hours that my daughter was in labor, menus were provided to her husband and me, so we didn't have to leave the room to scavenge for food.

This wasn't a run-of-the-mill pregnancy and delivery either. My daughter was having twins which were term (due the week she delivered) and thus her pregnancy was automatically considered high-risk. Fortunately, the obstetrician gathered us all together the day before and told us something one rarely hears a doctor say: "This is a journey and we can do it together. It may take time, but together, we will deliver these babies safe and sound." With that supportive, positive, and caring attitude, we all felt my daughter was safe and in good hands.

The rest of the hospital staff only added to the commitment. The nurses caring for my daughter made her feel safe; they never flinched when surprises occurred or hinted that anything was cause for concern. With every changing shift, a new nurse—full of vitality and passion for her work—came in and added to the positive energy in the room and our feeling of trust and confidence only grew. During the long hours of labor, the anesthesiologist who placed the epidural made sure to check in frequently, clearly concerned that my daughter remain as comfortable as possible. The obstetrician himself was omnipresent. In fact, you would never have guessed it was a regular workday for him and he was seeing other patients in his office, just five minutes from the maternity ward. When it was time to go to the delivery room, gently and with the utmost kindness, the doctor and staff guided and coached my daughter, her husband, and me through the most memorable experience of our lives; the welcoming of two beautiful twin girls into a calm and peaceful world.

The next two days spent in the hospital were nothing short of magical. Kindness, care, and support for mother and babies overflowed. Even though his main job was done, my daughter's obstetrician came to see us daily, spending literally hours providing confident and knowledgeable advice and reassurance. That is what I call excellent hospital care, where doctor and patient join forces to create a positive experience and outcome. Fact is, things do work out under these circumstances.

Our experience with Dr. Bitran at Mt. Sinai gives me hope for our hospital system; hope that it *does* have the potential to evolve into something wonderful. But all of us—physicians, nurses, administrators, trustees, public policy makers, and especially patients—are going to have to keep fighting and demanding change if it's really going to happen.

CHAPTER 7
SOLUTIONS: YOUR TURN TO CARRY THE BALL

"Today's medicine is at the end of its road. It can no longer be transformed, modified, readjusted. That's been tried too often. Today's medicine must DIE in order to be reborn. We must prepare its complete renovation."

—Maurice Delort

Over the past twenty-five years, since my awakening as a physician, I've devoured medical literature on a daily basis, including reading every ground-breaking book by other well-informed and well-researched critics of the healthcare system—many of them MDs like myself—all of whom, like me, have been beating the drums for change. With so many educated, informed insiders railing against the system, why are we still worse than ever?

I believe it's because there's a missing player out here in the field—that star quarterback who has been benched by the system, but who isn't even aware s/he should be in the game.

That player, of course, is you—the all-important patient.

You are the one who is going to carry that ball over the final goal line. It may be a very long game, indeed, but if you join us—and if we don't settle for less than we all deserve—together we will win.

I wanted to write this book as a prescription for a paradigm shift in healthcare—a shift in which you become the newest but most avid crusader on the frontlines for change. But it's not going to happen the way society has convinced you it should—by joining those feel-good "walks for the cure" with pink or red or purple ribbons on your shirt; or by paying $5.00 for a plastic wrist band to show your commitment to fighting for cures; or by donating that extra dollar at the checkout register of your grocery story to your local children's hospital. I hope some of the things you've learned in this book will inspire you to read more about the economics of medicine and medical research, which I promise will provide further evidence that few of these ways of "contributing" do little more than add to the hundreds of millions of dollars in compensation reaped by insurance, pharmaceutical, medical equipment companies and hospital CEOs—at the expense of both your wallet and, more importantly, your health.

I'm an immigrant to this country. I love America and believe fully in the American Dream—that everyone who works hard can achieve success and happiness. But health care is one area in which profit-seeking-run-amok is not only enriching the few, it is harming and even killing the many. It's time that you, the patient, had an honest and realistic bill of rights to help protect yourself from an impersonal system that doesn't care about you:

THE PATIENT'S MANIFESTO:

- *I am a human being, equally worthy of respect and dignity as any doctor I may consult.*
- *I am an adult who can and will make my own health care decisions.*
- *I will no longer allow any doctor or healthcare worker to treat me like a child.*
- *I acknowledge that medical issues and decisions can be very scary. I will commit to putting my fear aside when I am weighing my healthcare options. I will not rush to make any decisions when I am feeling emotional, confused, or fearful.*

- *I will designate a reliable advocate to represent me should I feel too ill or confused to represent myself.*
- *I don't need to be a doctor to understand—or to be able to learn—basic and even advanced concepts about my health and health conditions for me to make informed medical choices.*
- *There are no stupid questions when it comes to my health. If I ask a question and get a medical jargon answer, or am treated disrespectfully, I have the right to continue to ask for explanations until I get one I can understand. If I don't I will walk out and seek help elsewhere.*
- *I have the right and you (the entire membership of the healthcare delivery system) have the obligation to tell me the truth and not underplay possible side-effects or dangers of pharmaceuticals, treatments, procedures or tests you advise I undergo.*
- *I have the right to request second and even third opinions. I will not let fear of "hurting my doctor's feelings" dissuade me from seeking them. I will also seek different perspectives.*
- *I have the right to refuse any medication or treatment course I believe isn't right for me.*
- *I understand the doctor doesn't live in my body, thus can never understand how I feel, and it is my responsibility to make the final decision about my care.*
- *I have the obligation to listen to my own body and—even if it's contrary to what a doctor may be telling me—the ultimate decision for my own course of care or treatment is entirely my own.*
- *I have the right to decide what type of care I should get or refuse care. I will never allow a doctor to intimidate or bully me ever again.*

- *This is my life and my body. No one else but I have the right to decide what I should do.*

DEMANDING BETTER FROM YOUR DOCTORS

Taking control of your health begins first with making the right choices for your own life and second with your relationship with your doctors. After reading this book, I hope you understand that no patient can afford to believe the "doctor knows best" adage. Even if it's not the fault of the individual doctor—even if you have a doctor who is wonderful, well-trained and who genuinely cares—the system is so broken that you still cannot turn over complete control of your health and your life. No doctor can or should hold dominion over you. Remember, even the best doctors in the world are still victims of the various impersonal and greedy institutions that make up modern health care in the United States; institutions that should be here to protect us all, but which instead serve special interests —not yours.

The sad truth is, most people turn emotionally into little children when we visit our doctors. We surrender responsibility to someone who, in too many cases, speaks to us while barely looking up from a chart or computer. Why do we accept shoddy treatment from doctors when our bodies and our health are at stake? It's no longer a choice, but mandatory that we take ownership of our health and our care.

It's time to finally grow up.

How do you know a doctor is right for you? You would probably think the first step is checking her credentials. By all means, make sure you aren't dealing with a fraud. Make sure the doctor is licensed in the state in which s/he is practicing and go to the national database to check his/her malpractice records. However, even if a doctor has a number of malpractice suits you need to put them in proper perspective. Certain specialties are subject to a higher rate of malpractice suits and certain doctors tend to patients who are more litigious than others. For instance, ob-gyn is a specialty in which lawsuits are rampant. Everyone wants a perfect baby and if they don't get one they rush to blame the doctor. Surgical specialties are also high-risk. Wherever there is the possibility of permanent damage lawsuits are sure to follow. So there are other important factors to take into consideration.

Look for consistency. If a doctor stays in one place for most of his career, doesn't move from state to state, is known in the community and respected by patients, that is a very good sign. Belonging to medical societies, such as the AMA, or the staff of a hospital does not necessarily make for a good doctor. It may show s/he is involved and participates in the medical community and is likely to follow the party line, but it doesn't mean the doctor is right for you. Board certification in the specialty the doctor is practicing is important. However, it doesn't carry the weight it did twenty years ago. As medical fields are splitting open and more physicians are leaving the conventional, traditional way of thinking and practicing, many physicians who are trained in one specialty work in another, leaving their board certification behind. For example, there is no approved conventional specialty board in preventive medicine, so many of us practicing in this field are left to choose between conventional internal or alternative medicine, neither of which reflect the correct skills needed to practice prevention.

Since we started our not-for-profit organization in 2007, BHIonline.org my colleagues and I have trained many gynecologists, internists, psychiatrists, anesthesiologists, family practitioners—most board certified in these specialties—all lacking the proper training to provide preventive and integrated care their patients are seeking. Integrative, preventive, and bio-identical hormone training doesn't exist in any conventional specialty so an interested physician has to look outside their specialty.

There are thousands of physicians around the country that have broadened their practice scope and moved beyond their original specialty to learn how to do cosmetic procedures. Once the exclusive domain of dermatologists and plastic surgeons, Botox, fillers, and lasers are now part of many conventional doctors' menu of services. You have no way of determining if the doctor is good at these procedures or is just adding them to make extra money.

Most really good doctors still get their patients through word of mouth. Before doctors were permitted to advertise directly to the public, before insurance companies dominated health care and directed patients to their roster of participating physicians, patients chose their primary care practitioners because their friends and family endorsed a particular doctor's care and they lived in geographic proximity.

Today you only go to recommended doctors if you have the financial means to do so. Since most people are forced into health care dictated by insurance companies, most patients don't have a choice. Unless you are fortunate enough to be directed to a doctor in your plan by word of mouth, you will most likely have to choose blindly from a list of hundreds of participating doctors. Many medical practices are large and impersonal. There is a very small chance you will develop a substantial relationship with any doctor. Even if you find a doctor you like, chances are that by next year your insurance won't be working with the same group. For that reason alone you must take your Patient's Manifesto seriously and realize you alone can represent your best interests.

And please do not waste too much time on the Best Doctors lists and publications. They may help raise your awareness about certain specialists but too often they are tied into the hospitals who advertise in these publications.

All this information must serve you in a very positive way. It gives you the information and confidence to take control of your own health. How freeing and honest!

While you and I may not be able to change the system as a whole, you *can* change how the system works for you by changing your personal perspective. If you must use the system, use it with a new attitude. Regardless of how long you will be in a particular doctor's care, remember *you* are in charge. If you can choose a doctor, interview him or her before blindly deciding to follow his advice.

Think of your initial consultation with a new doctor as a job interview, where the doctor is the candidate for the job. If the doctor is willing to talk to you before you become a patient you're onto something. If that's not an option, move on. If the doctor agrees to meet with you, pay attention to how s/he behaves.

Here are some key factors for your "hiring" checklist:

1. *How does the doctor address you?* Respect is crucial and how the doctor addresses you is very telling. Stay away from doctors who call women "honey" or "dear." It is disrespectful and puts you in an inferior position.

2. *Does the doctor make eye contact with you?* Unless the doctor looks you right in the eye, with kindness and respect, you must move on. If s/he doesn't make eye contact s/he's doesn't see you as a human being and will be treating you as a blood test, condition or body part. That is dangerous.

3. *Does the doctor let you talk—and does she actually listen?* All the information you bring to the doctor or fill out in the office is important as baseline for your medical record, but cannot replace an open dialogue between you and your doctor. The first time you meet sets the foundation for the rest of the relationship. You need a doctor who listens to what you have to say. A doctor who cares to understand who you are.

4. *Does the doctor ask you questions about you and your family? Your job?*

5. *Both physicians and patients have been indoctrinated that our personal lives are relevant only to the therapist.* Nothing could be further from the truth. Everything that happens to you affects your health. No part of you operates independently. If the doctor doesn't ask personal questions, s/he will never be able to provide the correct treatment you need as an individual.

6. *Does your doctor encourage you to ask questions, without making you feel stupid for doing so?* There is no such thing as a stupid question. I cannot tell you how often patients preface their questions with, "I'm sorry doctor, please forgive me for asking a stupid question…" We have been conditioned by the arrogance of the medical profession to think we are less important than the doctor, hence our questions are stupid. If a doctor looks down his nose at you, ignores your questions, or answers you in an annoyed, condescending tone, you have to move on. This type of interaction will only hurt you.

7. *Does your doctor spend enough time with you? Does the visit with the doctor help you feel better?* The average primary care doctor visit is less than ten minutes. The median is 15.7 minutes.[59] In clinics and most insurance-run medical care settings, the average primary care doctor, internist, gynecologist and pediatrician are pushed to see between thirty and fifty patients a day. Any human being with common sense knows this is insane. How can a doctor take care of you with such ridiculous constraints on his/her time? And why would any patient allow him/herself to be a part of this assembly line type of care? If you don't feel your visit with the doctor has helped you feel better, you are seeing the wrong doctor.

You may think there is no way to change the status quo of assembly line medicine. There is and you have a very important role in bringing about change.

To correct this disaster we have two options:

1. **The doctor leaves.** Refusing to treat patients inhumanely, the doctor decides to leave this environment. You may think doctors rarely leave, but that isn't the case. Many get burned out and change professions altogether, while some look for jobs where insurance and the bottom line aren't the driving force.

2. **You—the patient—leave.** Once you understand there is no way you can get good care when a doctor acts like they're doing you a favor by spending six minutes with you, you have to take ownership of your life and walk out. You are better off with no health care than the inhumane type of care that has become the norm in our country today.

A doctor friend of mine, Peter, told me this dramatic story that I hope helps you take control of your health as well:

"DEAD WITHIN MONTHS"

Rebecca, Peter's cousin, was diagnosed with cancer. Through connections, Rebecca was able to get an appointment to see Dr. L—the top expert in her particular type of cancer—at the leading cancer hospital in New York City. Peter decided to go with her to provide moral support and lend a professional ear. He didn't tell the specialist he was a doctor; he just introduced himself by his first name. Together, Peter and Rebecca sat across the huge mahogany desk in Dr. L's office, while the famous cancer specialist reviewed her records. Once finished, Dr. L told Rebecca she was in luck because he was heading an exclusive clinical trial with a highly promising investigative new drug for her type of cancer he could get her into right away. When she started asking questions about her absolute risk and details of the clinical trial, Dr. L shot back that the science only addressed relative risk and her questions reflected her lack of scientific understanding. Dr. L didn't have time to waste with this annoying and nosey patient. He matter-of-factly told her that unless she entered his trial, the statistics on her cancer unequivocally showed she would be dead within three months.

Peter could no longer stay quiet. He asked Dr. L why he was scaring Rebecca and why it was so important for her to participate in this particular clinical trial. Defiantly, Dr. L turned the sheets with Rebecca's lab results to face Peter saying sarcastically with a sneer, "Okay, you read it and figure it out. I'm sure you know how to read lab results."

Peter took his cousin by the hand and left the doctor's office, never to return.

He found Rebecca another oncologist—one who was respectful and kind. Together, they decided on a course of treatment that both Rebecca and her doctor felt comfortable with. A course of treatment specifically designed for Rebecca.

Eight years later, Rebecca's cancer is long gone and she's doing just fine.

This is not a unique story, but it can become the rule on how doctors must behave and the system changes once patients take their power back.

THE NEW BREED OF DOCTOR

Finally, the great news:

In the past two decades a new breed of doctor has started to emerge. This doctor, though traditionally trained, cares about patients on a human level—as complete individuals, not just a collection of cells, organs, tests, and diseases. This new doctor is moving towards individualized, patient-centric care because it is only with this perspective on the patient and health care that true prevention and real healing can take place.

There are doctors coming up through the ranks, in both traditional medical schools and osteopathic schools, who really want to be your respectful partner. There are thousands already in practice who, like me, have become disillusioned with the current system but haven't given up on being good doctors; and thousands more, hungry for more training in prevention and patient-centric medicine outside the confines of the classical allopathic medical school training. These doctors—though they are trained in the statistics of relative-versus-absolute risk, test-and-treat mentality, and develop-a-drug- then create a disease—are caring and honest. They will recommend acupuncture, massage, and meditation before prescribing narcotics, blood pressure meds, or statins. These are doctors who understand the connection between stress, diet, nutrition, exercise, and health—and will address those details before sending their patients for tests. They are the doctors who, when presented with a lower back problem, will refer you to a progressive physical therapist who will teach you how to stretch and build core strength, long before rushing you off to get and MRI or sending you to a surgeon trained with the "when in doubt, cut it out" philosophy.

These new doctors are not looking *for* disease; we are working at *preventing* diseases and keeping you fearless and empowered.

Unfortunately, although it is clear that the present system doesn't work, conventional medicine still tries to discourage this kind of doctor.

You'll no doubt have read the myriad articles by old-school doctors trying to pigeonhole those who question the status quo as "quacks" and outliers. Look at what happened to Dr. Mehmet Oz. Whatever you may think of the hype that sometimes muddies the content of his television show, his more than twenty-year record as an outstanding cardiac surgeon, the hundreds of lives he has saved, and his attempt to enlighten and help Americans to take better care of themselves, stand on their own merits. Nearly two full years after Dr. Oz had been chastised for recommending a weight loss supplement with over-enthusiastic language on his show, suddenly—seemingly out of the blue—a group of "respected" academic doctors sent a letter to Columbia University, denouncing Dr. Oz as a quack and demanding he be fired from the academic institution. What the media didn't tell you was that the timing was no coincidence. In fact, Dr. Oz had spoken out on his show about the growing scientific evidence of serious health dangers from the multiplying GMOs (Genetically Modified Organisms) in our food supply. Why would such a simple statement make Dr. Oz a target?

The fight against GMOs has been waging for decades, largely ignored by the American media, despite the fact that in Europe, stringent laws have been put in place since 2007 to protect consumers against these foods. Here, the debate has been largely confined to the fringes of activism: progressives, consumer advocates, and the educated agricultural food science community. Dr. Oz, however, is watched by millions of "mainstream" Americans who may never have heard of GMOs and their potential dangers. Is it any coincidence that the doctors spearheading the campaign against him here on the payroll of Monsanto, the biggest producer and lobbyist for GMO's in the world? Having read this book, you now understand that the Vioxx scandal, the introduction of fraudulent scientific articles in mainstream peer reviewed medical journals, were just examples—the tip of a massive iceberg—of ways giant corporations endanger lives in the quest for profits. It sounds like a cliché, but usually the answers come easy once you "follow the money."

I'm not saying there aren't new-age quacks out there. Of course there are. Just be mindful to do your research in order to separate the true quacks from the mavericks, those who dare speak out and challenge the status quo.

The best way to silence an adversary is to destroy his or her credibility.

Don't forget what happened to Dr. Semelweiss who saved the lives of thousands of women by simply teaching his colleagues to wash their hands before delivering babies. He was fired from his job by doctors whose egos stood in the way of progress, leaving thousands of innocent women to die needlessly for years. Remember also that it was traditional academic medicine directly responsible for the tens of thousands of deaths from Vioxx and Celebrex and contaminated gastroscopes as well as the hundreds of thousands of deaths from hospital infections and medical mistakes. Be careful to look at every case individually, consider the evidence, and keep your mind open. You will find hidden villains— and heroes—in places you might never expect.

PROTECTING YOURSELF FROM HOSPITALS

"But I Need Surgery…"

In Chapter 6, you learned all the reasons to stay away from hospitals. Of course, that's not always possible. If you need surgery you have to go to the hospital. Here are some tools that will help you make wiser and safer decisions.

- **More than a second opinion, you need a second *perspective*.** Doctors who have similar training have similar opinions. While some surgeons may be quicker to operate than others, in general you can be fairly sure a surgeon will recommend surgery. Indeed, some surgeons are more adept than others so choosing the best one you will improve your chances for a great outcome. Also, the best surgeon is the one with the most experience in the particular surgical procedure you need so find that doctor! Before the decision to operate has been made, seek a different perspective from a doctor with different kind of training. For instance, for a heart ailment, you might visit a conventional cardiologist, an integrative internist, as well as a holistic doctor who will see you as the whole person, not just a heart. A fresh perspective is a more evolved take on the traditional second opinion, and will go a long way in providing better information and more appropriate care.

- **Ask why the procedure is necessary.** Be sure you understand and are totally clear how this surgery will correct your problem. When the doctor reassures you this is the best way to proceed, you may want to take some time to do research on your own. The goal of your research shouldn't be to scare you more, but rather to find balance. Keep in mind that surgery, biopsy, and any invasive procedure will change your body's anatomy and immune system forever. *Once you take it out you can never put it back in.*

- **Doctors will always give you statistics to strengthen their argument.** A gynecologist told one of my patients, a forty-five-year-old woman with an ovarian cyst, that she had a "10 percent chance of cancer." Why not tell her there was a 90 percent chance the cyst was benign? Sure, the doctor was honest but why put a negative spin on the information? My patient opted for surgery because she was scared of being one of the 10 percent. The truth is, no doctor and no statistic can ever predict what the future holds or what your personal odds of dying or getting a certain disease are. We are individuals, not statistics.

- **Don't believe the aftermath of surgery is going to be a breeze.** There is no such thing as no side-effects and recovery is never easy, no matter what you are told. For optimal outcomes, you need a team of doctors who know how to treat you before and after surgery, help improve your recovery, and ease your return back to your regular life.

- **Find out the risks and complications of having the operation.** Even the smallest of surgeries contains risks. Be sure you understand what they are and what, if anything, you can do to minimize those risks. Ask if there is any reason the risks might be greater in your case (for instance, if you have diabetes or other chronic illness). Make sure the surgeon knows your entire medical history and confers with your other primary doctor(s) so you don't become a statistic.

- **Know the difference between absolute and relative risk.** When a doctor talks about risk, it's always about relative risk. That doesn't really apply to you. It is a way to massage scientific data to scare you into taking action. *Relative risk* is a way of comparing risks to figure out how much more likely one is compared to the other. *Absolute risk* is the actual risk of something happening to you. By the definitions alone it becomes clear there is no way any doctor can ever tell you what your absolute risk is. That is why you can't just accept statistical mumbo jumbo as factual information that pertains to you.

- **Do your own research.** Use websites like www.consumerreportshealth.org and www.hospitalcompare.hhs.com to look for ratings of hospitals in your area. While most patients like to follow their doctors and go to whatever hospital the doctor is affiliated with, many doctors are on staff at more than one hospital. Ask people who have had similar surgeries and worked with the doctor of your choice about their experiences. No matter how routine your procedure may be, it's life altering for you, so don't be cavalier about your operation. Get all the facts you can.

- **If you're a patient in a hospital, make sure everyone who enters your room—from doctors and nurses to your visitors—washes their hands.** Hand-washing is the single most effective defense against infection.

- **People who don't speak up are more likely to become statistics.** The squeaky wheel story applies to medical care more than you think. We are talking about the rest of your life here. Don't become a faceless, nameless person in the crowd. People justify inexcusable behavior. "He's the best surgeon, so I don't really care how he treats me. All he has to do is perform the surgery well." As for the doctor, he's got his own set of excuses: "Bedside manner is just another old wives tale." "It's all about how excellent I am technically." Don't believe it for a minute. No matter how famous or talented your physician is, if the doctor doesn't treat you with care and respect, your life is at risk.

- **Bring someone with you when you're asking the doctor questions.** Even under normal circumstances, when people go to the doctor for routine exams, they can't remember what the doctor said out of fear. When you're ill and under stress, things get much worse. Ask a supportive friend or loved one to come with you and take notes. Don't be embarrassed to tell the doctor if you don't understand or need her to repeat something s/he said. Since all the doctor visits are about you and your health, you must stand up for yourself and pay attention. And you don't have to agree to anything immediately. Unless you are having emergency surgery, you have time to figure it out and come back with your decision later. Don't allow the doctor to pressure you to decide then and there.

- **Make sure you pay attention to the anesthesiologist.** A patient of mine, Margot, was having elective surgery. The night before, after she had begun her fast and the other pre-surgical rituals she'd been instructed to follow, the anesthesiologist called her at home. While her surgeon had only asked about the prescription medications Margot was on, the anesthesiologist made her go to her kitchen cabinet and read through every supplement she was taking. As it turned out, a "metabolic enhancer" for weight loss that Margot's trainer had recommended had been shown in studies to be risky to the heart under general anesthesia. The anesthesiologist was up to date on her science, and didn't want Margot, though young and healthy to take the risk. She insisted that Margot stop taking the supplement and reschedule her surgery. Though it was a huge inconvenience to be sure, it was the kind of prudent action that the best physicians will always insist on taking for the safety of the patient.

Margot might not have had to reschedule her surgery at the last minute if she'd demanded answers to the following questions:

- Do you need to stop taking your medications, herbal supplements, or over-the-counter drugs?
- Is there anything you can do to ensure a smoother recovery process? (E.g., hydrate, get a significant amount of sleep the night before, take arnica montana to prevent bruising, supplements to help heal faster, etc.)
- Should you fast before the surgery? For how many hours?
- How long, approximately will the surgery take?
- What about post-op hospital stay? In-home recovery?

The best doctors provide very specific instructions and encourage you to be involved at every step of the process to make sure your surgery and recovery are successful.

- **Never accept vague answers.** The more concrete the answer, the more likely the doctor has actually paid attention to your question. This information may all be in the fine print on the consent form you sign, but few patients will read every page and fully understand what you're getting into. A doctor who cares about you will talk to you, human to human, prepare you to the best of his/her ability, and allay your fears about the procedure.

- **The doctor will visit you after surgery.** Make sure your surgeon will remember you after the surgery and come in to see you every day you are in the hospital and stay as available to you as before the surgery.

FIGHTING THE CULTURE OF "HEALTH SCARE"

I hope you'll take the information in this book—the truth, some of it not so easy to accept, from my forty years of being a doctor—and put it to good use right away. Even if you suffer with an accurately diagnosed illness, disease, or condition, why not try to avoid thinking of yourself as that disease? Work at changing your inner voice; instead of thinking "my disease" think "my health." Think of disease as a temporary, uninvited visitor. You don't have to keep listening to all the pharmaceutical ads that try to scare you, or say yes to any doctor who over tests you to death.

A brilliant palliative care doctor, helping Melissa cope with her ninety-one-year old father's death, said something that every doctor (and patient) should remember: "Death is not the enemy. Suffering is."

Recognizing our own mortality is frightening but it's also empowering. Some of us live longer than others; some of us lead healthier lives than others. Each one of us must decide what we want to do with our life. Is life simply about surviving; going from one drug to another or one invasive test to another, looking for diseases that might not even be there? Or is it about living a productive life of high quality, no matter how long we're here for?

At the end of the day none of us—neither doctors nor patients—know when our last day on earth will be or what will bring about our demise.

We are not God. We are all the same. Doctors may have skills you may need on certain occasions. But that's about all they are.

It's your life and you need to decide to live it on your terms.

A NEW KIND OF DOCTOR'S OFFICE—YOUR REFUGE FROM FEAR

Can you imagine looking forward to a visit to your doctor's office because it was actually a calming place; a refuge from fear?

Imagine that. How many doctors do you know whose offices are a place of calm and kindness? Where receptionists greet you with a smile and know your name and ask about your family and ask if you'd like a cold drink rather than demanding your insurance card without looking up from the computer screen? Where you sit in a clean, comfortable chair and leaf through a variety of new, crisp magazines? What if you looked around you in the soothing, golden light and saw walls of appealing colors, peppered with interesting and inspiring artwork, accompanied by relaxing music playing softly in the background? I'm not describing a spa; I'm describing a real doctor's office.

And what about the doctor? How many of you can honestly say you are looking forward to seeing your doctor because when you leave his or her office, you feel thoroughly informed, reassured, empowered, fearless, and ready to take on the world and enjoy your life?

As the famous line in *Field of Dreams* goes, "If you build it, they will come," it's high time we start building. Don't accept less than the best medical care you deserve. Find that doctor whose office is a safe haven of kindness, support, and even love for you. See how much better you will do.

This is the best evidence-based medicine anyone needs. Evidence based on the most important person there is—you.

As I did a few pages back for the patient, I'd like to propose a new manifesto for our new breed of doctor—a new promise we make to our patients that goes above and beyond our Hippocratic Oath:

THE DOCTOR'S MANIFESTO

- *I will take my Hippocratic Oath to "first, do no harm" seriously.*
- *I will never take myself too seriously!*
- *I will eliminate arrogance from my personality.*
- *I will take my own ego out of the examination room and out of my interactions with patients and other medical professionals.*
- *I will respect and care for each one of my patients to the best of my abilities as a human being.*
- *I will listen to my patients.*
- *I will honestly and caringly, without judgment or preconceived notions, do my best to understand each of my patients—not just the results of their tests—and put everything into context with the details of their lives.*
- *I will respect my patients and view them as the complex human beings they are, not collections of organs, conditions, or diseases.*
- *I will communicate with each patient with full transparency, sharing complete information to the best of my ability. I will speak to my patients in a language they can understand and not hide behind medical jargon.*

- *I will never make a patient feel stupid or inferior in any way. I will answer as many questions as the patient requires to feel comfortable and well informed.*
- *I will never make my patient feel bad or guilty for seeking a second opinion.*
- *I will open my mind to another professional's perspective and learn to consider other opinions as resources that can help me become a better doctor.*
- *I will respect other doctors and openly and kindly communicate and collaborate with them in order to improve the care we give to our patients.*
- *I won't use derogatory terms to refer to other doctors' recommendations.*
- *I won't assume I have the "only" right answer when it comes to treating a patient.*
- *I will always put my patients' best interests ahead of any other considerations.*
- *I will respect and understand that my patient's life, body, and health belong to him/her, and that s/he is the ultimate authority on the choices s/he makes for him/herself.*
- *I will never bully or scare patients into following my advice.*
- *I will strive to make my office a place of solace and kindness for the patient.*
- *I will do my part in eliminating fear from health care.*

EPILOGUE
THE EMPOWERED PATIENT

"The art of medicine consists of amusing the patient while nature cures the disease."

—Voltaire

Every journey begins with a first step and for many it will not be an overnight transformation from *perfect patient* to *empowered patient*. I hope, however, that the information contained in this book has started that process for you. My goal in presenting a comprehensive and honest look at the present state of our healthcare system is to help you make sense of a very disjointed picture. When you read or watch the news, you may hear of terrible things happening in one sector or another of health care, but there is no one helping you connect the dots. Not being able to put the pieces together, keeps you trapped in victim mode when your turn comes to enter the system.

I hope what you've read here gives you pause. Remember that there's more to health care than meets the eye. Maybe you'll think twice before regressing into the role of perfect patient. Maybe you'll take ownership of your life and refuse to be bullied by arrogance and greed. Ultimately, I hope you choose to live your life free of fear.

This idea of the empowered patient isn't new. In fact, the patient-as-victim model of health care didn't happen overnight, it took many decades to develop so it will take a long time to correct.

The following is a true story from a time when, even more than today, patients (particularly women) were expected to keep their mouths shut and obey their doctors without question. Given the "dark ages" in which these events occurred, the woman at their center was a symbol of self-confidence and courage.

BABETTE ROSMOND'S STORY[60]

In February of 1971, Babette Rosmond, a forty-nine-year old magazine editor and author living in Manhattan, discovered an olive-sized lump in her breast. When she entered a Manhattan hospital for a biopsy, Babette refused to sign a routine release, which stated that if the frozen section pathology report taken in the OR (while she was still under anesthesia) showed cancer, she gave permission to the surgeon to remove her breast. Two of her friends had undergone radical mastectomies and the details of their physical and emotional ordeals were sad and horrific. In a radical mastectomy, the breast, underarm lymph nodes, and chest wall muscles on the side of the cancer are removed, leaving the woman with a hollow chest wall and lymphedema (permanently swollen arm and hand).

The report showed the tumor to be cancer, but Ms. Rosmond refused surgery and made it clear that she needed time before making such a life-changing decision. Her doctor's reaction was far from compassionate. He spoke to her as if she was an errant child and angrily told her that without the surgery, she would be dead in three weeks. She left that doctor's "care" and, using her talent as an experienced investigative journalist, sought out one who would listen to her, respect her as an equal, and discuss her options with her as an adult.

She found such a doctor in Dr. George Crile Jr., of the Cleveland Clinic, who at the time was challenging the medical community and making waves with his research, proving that when breast cancer is small and localized, radical mastectomies were unnecessary. After working hand in hand with Babette to get her up to speed with the findings of his research and helping her weigh her choices by laying out their pros and cons, they agreed on a partial mastectomy. The surgery was successful, but afterward Ms. Rosmond once again had to take control of her treatment, and she declined Dr. Crile's suggestion for localized radiation.

Rosamond documented her experience of battling with the (mostly male) medical establishment in her book, The Invisible Worm: A Woman's Right to Choose an Alternate to Radical Surgery. *She appeared on television shows including,* The David Susskind Show. *During that appearance, she held her own against Dr. Jerome Urban of Memorial Sloan Kettering Hospital, a staunch proponent of radical surgery. She made her position very clear: she wasn't urging women to have her procedure. Her crusade was for women's rights to be informed of all their medical options, so they could make adult decisions based on facts, not on what some doctor orders them to do.*

Ms. Rosmond died in 1997 at the age of seventy-five. The breast cancer never recurred.

The story of Babette Rosmond is inspiring and rare. I chose to include it in this book because it has given hope to so many. She certainly was a pioneer in the 1970s. Surprisingly, today too many women and men still live in the mindset of forty years ago and continue to allow the system and its doctors to bully them into making decisions that, too often, ruin their lives.

Throughout this book, you've read stories from the life of my patient, Victoria Reggio. I have been blessed to watch her transformation from passive spectator in her own life to proactive owner of both her health and happiness.

I wanted to end this book with some final words from her on becoming an "empowered patient"—and person.

CHOICES, CROSSROADS, CONSEQUENCES

The alarm goes off in the morning and we face our first choice of the day. Do we get up and take on the challenges of life or do we roll over and go back to sleep?

When we face the day at work, we are confronted with more choices. Should we eat that gooey Danish pastry sitting on the coffee cart, or spend a few extra minutes preparing oatmeal with fruit in the office kitchen? Should we shovel down a fast-food burger while we spend our lunch hour hunched over our computers, or take a brisk fifteen-minute walk outside then fuel our bodies with a salad and some lean protein? Should we go home to "unwind" with a few glasses of wine and a sodium-filled frozen dinner, or pour a refreshing green tea over ice and stir fry some fresh vegetables with protein, and a whole grain, like quinoa or brown rice?

If our choices result in our being overweight, sluggish, depressed and unproductive, it's time to examine our lifestyle and consider this a crossroad to changing our lives.

I'll use myself as an example. After a stressful childhood and adolescence, I graduated from college and entered the competitive world of a struggling actress. I supported myself by working full time for a magazine. Of course, like many twenty-somethings I did a lot of partying. Sleep was something I squeezed in…occasionally. This exhaustive physical and emotional roller coaster went off the rails when I was diagnosed with cancer. While hospitalized, attached to all sorts of tubes and wires, I had a lot of time to think about the choices I had made. I knew that I had reached the first major crossroad in my life. I never wanted to be flat on my back again, helpless and wondering if I was going to live or die. I decided it was time to take control of my life. That meant taking control of my health.

As I recovered, I researched nutrition and started a regular schedule of exercise. Getting enough sleep became a top priority, so I consumed no alcohol

Monday through Friday. A glass of wine might have given me the sense of relaxation and I would even fall into a deep sleep only to wake up at 2:00 a.m. because I was missing the first and important stage of REM (rapid eye movement) sleep. When I researched sleep deprivation, I learned that, according to the Centers for Disease Control (CDC), 30 percent of American workers are sleep-deprived.

For me, the benefits of becoming more sleep conscious were immediate. I was more alert, happier, and looked better. I lost weight by not wasting calories on alcohol. "Happy hour" was now the time I spent at the gym. Of course, not everyone can afford or have access to a gym membership, and for some people, it's simply not enjoyable. If that seems too intense, the great outdoors is free. There is no better exercise than a brisk, refreshing walk. Don't just attend your kids' sporting events; play with them as well. There are so many gym-free alternatives that won't break the bank and will keep you fit and flexible.

But taking charge of your health is about more than just diet, exercise, and sleep. It's about taking back your power. One of the most important things my run-in with cancer taught me was the very important word, "no." I stopped politely giving in to many of the demands that others were placing on my life. There was a paradigm shift; I could love my friends, family, and my work—without sacrificing my health for them.

When Dr. Erika talks about the "empowered patient," I'm proud that she thinks of me as an example. If I can do it, you can too. Instead of joining the nation of people obsessed with reality television—watching others as they move along in their lives—it's time for you to do the most important work — create your own healthy reality.

I've watched Vicki for more than a decade now. She is smart, self-assured, and healthy. She's made tough decisions that have ultimately brought her health and personal satisfaction. Patients like Vicki are the ones who are changing health care for the better—because they won't accept anything less than the best. I know you too can become one of these empowered patients. It's easier than you think. Just remember that it's your life and you can choose not to live in fear. The rest will fall into place.

GLOSSARY

Academic Medical Center: A health care facility that is often linked to a medical school and/or university complex and closely affiliated with or part of a degree-granting university. Teaching of medical students and physicians in training; research; tertiary patient care. Additional components: Schools for other health professions – nursing, pharmacy, dentistry, allied health professions and other clinical entities, faculty group practices, community health centers, nursing homes and community-based networks of practitioners.

Actuarial Table: Table of statistical data.

Acute care: Branch of secondary health care where a patient receives active but short-term treatment for a severe injury or episode of illness, an urgent medical condition, or during recovery from surgery. In medical terms, care for acute health conditions is the opposite from chronic care, or long term care.

Adrenaline Rush: Sudden burst of energy from an increase in the hormone and neurotransmitter adrenaline, esp. increased heart rate and blood pressure, perspiration, blood sugar, and metabolism.

Affordable Care Act: The landmark health reform legislation passed by the 111th Congress and signed into law by President Barack Obama in March 2010.

Alkaline: Having the properties of an alkali, or containing alkali; having a pH greater than 7.

Allopathic medical school training: Allopathic means a system of medicine that uses agents (such as drugs or surgery) that produce effects different from those of the disease being treated (as opposed to homeopathic medicine).

Anatomy: The branch of science concerned with the bodily structure of humans, animals, and other living organisms, especially as revealed by dissection and the separation of parts.

Anemia: Condition marked by a deficiency of red blood cells or of hemoglobin in the blood, resulting in pallor and weariness.

Anesthesiologist: Physician trained in anesthesia and perioperative medicine.

Angiography (Angiogram): Examination by X-ray of blood or lymph vessels, carried out after introduction of a radiopaque substance.

Annual physical: Yearly wellness exam to review health status and create a plan for preventing disease and ensuring wellness.

Anti-inflammatory: Reducing inflammation swelling, tenderness, fever and pain.

A Priori: Relating to or denoting reasoning or knowledge that proceeds from theoretical deduction rather than from observation or experience.

Arteries: Any of the muscular-walled tubes forming part of the circulation system by which blood (mainly that which has been oxygenated) is conveyed from the heart to all parts of the body.

Arthroscopy: Procedure for diagnosing and treating joint problems. A surgeon inserts a narrow tube attached to a fiber-optic video camera through a small incision — about the size of a buttonhole. The view inside the joint is transmitted to a high-definition video monitor.

Asthma: A respiratory condition marked by spasms in the bronchi of the lungs, causing difficulty in breathing. It usually results from an allergic reaction or other forms of hypersensitivity.

Benign Fibroadenoma: The most common benign tumor of the breast. It is the most common breast tumor in women under age 30. A fibroadenoma is made up of breast gland tissue and tissue that helps support the breast gland tissue.

Biochemistry: The branch of science concerned with the chemical and physiochemical processes that occur within living organisms.

Bioidentical hormones: Estradiol, progesterone, testosterone, thyroid and adrenal hormones identical to the human hormones only pharmaceutically produced. Have the same effects as their human versions.

Biopsies: Sample of tissue taken from the body in order to examine it more closely.

Bipolar Depression: A mental disorder characterized by periods of elevated mood and periods of depression.

Black Death: One of the most devastating pandemics in human history, resulting in the deaths of an estimated 75 to 200 million people and peaking in Europe in the years 1346–53.

Blood clot: Gelatinous or semisolid mass of coagulated blood.

Bone marrow biopsy: Removal of marrow from inside bone. Bone marrow is the soft tissue inside bones that helps form blood cells.

Bronchitis: Inflammation of the mucous membrane in the bronchial tubes. It typically causes bronchospasm and coughing and may be caused by viruses, bacteria and allergies.

Cancer: Disease caused by an uncontrolled division of abnormal cells in the body.

Cardiac Surgery: Surgery on the heart and/or the proximal great vessels.

Cardiologist: Doctor with special training and skill in finding, treating diseases of the heart and blood vessels.

Catheter: Flexible tube inserted through a narrow opening into a body cavity, particularly the bladder, to remove fluid.

Cervical Cancer: A type of cancer that occurs in the cells of the cervix— the lower part of the uterus that connects to the vagina.

Chemotherapy: Treatment of disease by the use of chemical substances, especially the treatment of cancer with cytotoxic and other drugs.

Cholera: Infectious and often fatal bacterial disease of the small intestine typically contracted from infected water supplies and causing severe vomiting and diarrhea.

Coercive Persuasion: Theoretical indoctrination process which results in "an impairment of autonomy, an inability to think independently, and a disruption of beliefs and affiliations."

Collapsed lung: Condition in which the space between the wall of the chest cavity and the lung itself fills with air, causing all or a portion of the lung to collapse.

Colonoscopy: Exam used to detect changes or abnormalities in the large intestine (colon) and rectum. During a colonoscopy, a long, flexible tube (colonoscope) is inserted into the rectum and colon. A tiny video camera at the tip of the tube allows the doctor to view the inside of the entire colon. Biopsies and polyp removal can be performed through the tube.

Colposcopy: Diagnostic procedure to examine illuminate and magnified view of the cervix and the tissues of the vagina and vulva.

Consciousness: The state of being awake and aware of one's surroundings.

CPT (Current Procedural Terminology) codes: Medical code set that is used to report medical, surgical, and diagnostic procedures and services to entities such as physicians, health insurance companies and accreditation organizations.

Critical care: The specialized care of patients whose conditions are life-threatening and who require comprehensive care and constant monitoring, usually in intensive care units.

Depression: Feelings of severe despondency and dejection.

Diabetes: A metabolic disease in which the body's inability to produce any or enough insulin causes elevated levels of glucose in the blood and affects the entire body's normal function.

Diagnostic errors: Mistake in judgment regarding the cause of an illness.

Direct-to-consumer advertising (DTC advertising): Sometimes refers to the marketing of pharmaceutical products but applies in other areas as well. This form of advertising is directed toward patients, rather than healthcare professionals.

DMS (Diagnostic Statistical Manual of Mental Disorders): The standard classification of mental disorders used by mental health professionals in the United States.

EMR (Electronic Medical Record): A digital version of the traditional paper-based medical record for an individual. The EMR represents a medical record within a single facility, such as a doctor's office, hospital or a clinic.

Endoscopy suite: Dedicated area where medical procedures are performed with endoscopes, which are cameras used to visualize structures within the body, such as the digestive tract and genitourinary system.

Erectile Dysfunction: Inability of a man to maintain an erection sufficient for satisfying sexual activity.

Esophageal Perforation: Hole in the esophagus. The esophagus is the tube that food and liquids pass through on the way from mouth to stomach. Perforation of the esophagus is uncommon, but it is a serious medical condition

Evidence based medicine (EBM): Originally defined as the conscientious, explicit, and judicious use of current best evidence in making decisions about the care of individual patients.

Fertility Specialist: Physician who assists couples, and sometimes individuals, who want to become parents but for medical reasons have been unable to achieve this goal via the natural course

Fibroid: Benign tumor of muscular and fibrous tissues, typically found in the wall of the uterus.

Fibromyalgia: A chronic disorder characterized by widespread musculoskeletal pain, fatigue, and tenderness in localized areas.

Flu shot: An influenza vaccine administered by injection.

Gastric Motility: Gastrointestinal (GI) motility is defined by the movements of the digestive system and the transit of the contents within it. When nerves or muscles in any portion of the digestive tract do not function with their normal strength and coordination, a person develops symptoms related to motility problems.

Gastritis: Inflammation of the lining of the stomach.

Gastroenterologist: A physician who specializes in the diagnosis and treatment of diseases of the digestive system.

Genomics: Branch of molecular biology concerned with the structure, function, evolution, and mapping of genes.

Gynecologist: Physician who specializes in treating diseases of the female reproductive organs and providing well-woman health care that focuses primarily on the reproductive organs.

Heartburn: A form of indigestion felt as a burning sensation in the chest, caused by acid regurgitation into the esophagus.

Heart Disease: Generally refers to conditions that involve narrowed or blocked blood vessels that may lead to a heart attack, chest pain (angina) or stroke as well as heart conditions, such as those that affect heart muscle, valves or rhythm.

Hematology: Study of blood disorders: anemia, bleeding problems, etc.

Herd Mentality: Describes how people are influenced by their peers to adopt certain behaviors, follow trends, and/or purchase items.

High Blood Pressure (HBP): A serious condition that can lead to coronary heart disease, heart failure, stroke, kidney failure, and other health problems.

HMO: Health Maintenance Organization (HMO) is an organization that provides or arranges managed care for health insurance, self-funded health care benefit plans, individuals, and other entities in the United States and acts as a liaison with health care providers (hospitals, doctors, etc.) on a prepaid basis.

Hospital-acquired infections nosocomial infection: Infections acquired in hospitals and other healthcare facilities. To be classified as a nosocomial infection, the patient must have been admitted for reasons other than the infection.

Hot Flashes: Sudden feeling of feverish heat, typically a symptom of menopause.

HPV (Human Papillomavirus): A very common virus in men and women. It is passed on through genital contact, most often during vaginal and anal sex. Most sexually active people will get HPV at some time in their lives, though most will never know it because HPV usually has no signs or symptoms.

Hymen: Membrane that partially closes the opening of the vagina and whose presence is traditionally taken to be a mark of virginity.

Hysterectomy: Surgical procedure to remove the uterus but not the ovaries.

Ibuprofen: A synthetic compound used widely as an analgesic and anti-inflammatory drug

ICD (International Classification of Diseases): Medical code that defines the universe of diseases, disorders, injuries and other related health conditions. The insurance claim form ICD-9 or the newer ICD-10 coding system is a diagnostic code that reflects disease diagnosis. The CPT codes are specific for procedures performed. For instance: upper endoscopy, gastroscopy, biopsies of the esophagus and stomach, cultures of the stomach, just to name a few. DSM codes are for psychiatric illnesses.

Incentive Spirometer: A device given to patients after surgery to help improve respiratory function.

Inconclusive: Not leading to a firm conclusion; not ending doubt or dispute.

Indoctrination: Process of inculcating ideas, attitudes, cognitive strategies or a professional methodology. Indoctrination is a critical component in the transfer of cultures, customs, and traditions from one generation to the next.

Insomnia: Habitual sleeplessness; inability to sleep.

Internal medicine or general medicine: The medical specialty dealing with the diagnosis and treatment of adult diseases. Physicians specializing in internal medicine are called internists.

Invasive tests: Involve various forms of changing body integrity. Examples are inserting catheters into the blood vessels of the heart in order to get a closer look at the coronary arteries or to stimulate and test the electrical system of the heart, biopsies, aspirations of cysts, etc.

Lyme disease: An infectious disease characterized at first by a rash, headache, fever, and chills, and later by possible arthritis and neurological and cardiac disorders, caused by bacteria that are transmitted by deer ticks.

Lymphatic Drainage Therapy (LDT): Gentle, light-touch, noninvasive technique that offers qualified therapists a natural complement to their existing health care protocols.

Lymphoma: Cancer of the lymphatic system.

Malaria: Intermittent and remittent fever caused by a protozoan parasite that invades the red blood cells. The parasite is transmitted by mosquitoes in many tropical and subtropical regions.

Mammogram: An X-ray of the breast that is taken with a device that compresses and flattens the breast. A mammogram can help a health professional decide whether a lump in the breast is a gland, a harmless cyst, or a tumor.

Measles: An infectious viral disease causing fever and a red rash on the skin, typically occurring in childhood.

Medical College Admission Test: A computer-based standardized examination for prospective medical students in the United States, Australia and Canada.

Medical Industrial Complex: Made up of doctors, hospitals, nursing homes, nurses, physician assistants, aides, paramedical personnel, insurance companies, drug manufacturers, hospital supply and equipment companies, real estate and construction businesses, health systems consulting and accounting firms, advertising and marketing companies, media, and banks.

Menopause: Normal condition all women experience as they age. The term "menopause" can describe any of the changes a woman experiences before or after she stops menstruating. It marks the end reproductive cycle.

Microscope: Optical instrument used for viewing very small objects, such as mineral samples or animal or plant cells, typically magnified several hundred times.

MRI: Magnetic resonance imaging (MRI) is a test that uses a magnetic field and pulses of radio wave energy to obtain pictures of organs and structures inside the body. In many cases, MRI gives different information about structures in the body than can be seen on X-ray, ultrasound, or computed tomography (CT) scan.

MRSA Methicillin-resistant Staphylococcus aureus: A bacterium responsible for several difficult-to-treat infections in humans. It is also called oxacillin-resistant Staphylococcus aureus.

Multiple sclerosis: A chronic, typically progressive disease involving damage to the sheaths of nerve cells in the brain and spinal cord, whose symptoms may include numbness, impairment of speech and of muscular coordination, blurred vision, and severe fatigue.

Neuropathy: Disease or dysfunction of one or more peripheral nerves, typically causing numbness, weakness or loss of general neurologic function in the hands and feet.

NSAID (non-steroidal anti-inflammatories): A class of analgesic medication that reduces pain, fever and inflammation.

Nursing home: Private institution providing residential accommodations with health care, especially for elderly people.

Objective findings: Findings of disability that can be seen, felt, or measured by an examining physician.

Omnipotent: Having unlimited power; able to do anything.

Oncology: Study and treatment of tumors benign and cancerous.

Oophorectomy: Surgical removal of one or both ovaries; ovariectomy.

OTC (over-the-counter) medication: Are medicines sold directly to a consumer without a prescription, from a healthcare professional, as compared to prescription drugs, which may be sold only to consumers possessing a valid prescription.

Ovaries: Female reproductive organ in which ova or eggs are produced.

PAE Preventable or avoidable adverse events: Direct result of failure(s) to follow recognized, evidence-based best practices or guidelines at the individual and/or system level.

Pap Smear: A screening test for cervical cancer based on the examination of cells under the microscope. The cells are collected from the cervix, smeared on a slide and specifically stained to reveal premalignant (before cancer) and malignant (cancer) changes as well as changes due to noncancerous conditions such as inflammation from infections.

Paramedical Personnel: Personnel who assists physicians and nurses in their activities.

Pathology: The science of the causes and effects of diseases, especially the branch of medicine that deals with the laboratory examination of samples of body tissue for diagnostic or forensic purposes.

Patient safety: A new healthcare discipline that emphasizes the reporting, analysis, and prevention of medical error that often leads to adverse healthcare events.

Pediatrician: Medical practitioner specializing in children and their diseases.

Peer-review: The process of subjecting an author's scholarly work, research, or ideas to the scrutiny of others who are experts in the same field, before a paper describing this work is published in a journal or as a book.

Pericardial window: Surgical procedure to create an opening — or "window" — from the pericardial space to the pleural cavity used to drain fluid accumulated around the heart.

PET Scan: Type of imaging test. It uses a radioactive substance called a tracer to look for disease in the body. A PET scan shows how organs and tissues are working.

Pharmacology: The branch of medicine concerned with the uses, effects, and modes of action of drugs.

Physician assistants: Trained individuals who are certified to provide basic medical services (diagnosis and treatment of common ailments) usually under the supervision of a licensed physician—called also PA.

Physiology: The branch of biology that deals with the normal functions of living organisms and their parts.

PMS: Premenstrual syndrome (known as PMS) involves a variety of physical, mental, and behavioral symptoms tied to a woman's menstrual cycle. By definition, symptoms occur during the two weeks before a woman's period starts, known as the luteal phase of the menstrual cycle. The symptoms typically become more intense in the 2-3 days prior to the period and usually resolve after the first day or two of flow.

Pneumonia shot Pneumococcal vaccination: A method of preventing a specific type of lung infection (pneumonia) that is caused by pneumococcus bacterium. There are more than 80 different types of pneumococcus bacteria — 23 of them covered by the vaccine. The vaccine is injected into the body to stimulate immune system to produce antibodies that are directed against pneumococcus bacteria.

Preventive care medicine model: Relating to the branch of medicine concerned with prolonging life and preventing disease. Also known as Prevention and wellness medicine.

Prostate cancer: Cancer that occurs in a man's prostate — a small walnut-shaped gland that produces the seminal fluid that nourishes and transports sperm. Prostate cancer is one of the most common types of cancer in older men.

Proteomics: The study of proteomes (proteins expressed by genes) and their functions.

Protocols: Official procedures and systems of rules governing the practice of conventionally accepted medical care.

PSA: A protein produced by the prostate gland. A blood test for PSA may be used to screen for cancer of the prostate and to monitor treatment of the disease.

Psychiatry: Study and treatment of mental illness, emotional disturbance, and abnormal behavior.

Pulmonary arteries: The arteries carrying blood from the right ventricle of the heart to the lungs for oxygenation.

Pulmonary Embolus: Occurs when a blood clot blocks blood flowing through an artery that feeds the lungs. Typically, a blood clot first forms in an arm or leg (deep venous thrombosis or DVT) and then eventually breaks free and travels to the lungs.

Pulmonologist: A physician who possesses specialized knowledge and skill in the diagnosis and treatment of pulmonary (lung) conditions and diseases.

Pure Science: Science depending on deductions from demonstrated truths, such as mathematics or logic, or studied without regard to practical applications.

Quality of Life: The standard of health, comfort, and happiness experienced by an individual or group.

Radiation: Emission of energy as electromagnetic waves or as moving subatomic particles, especially high-energy particles that cause ionization. Used to treat various cancers.

Rehabilitation facility: Facility providing therapy and training for rehabilitation. The center may offer occupational therapy, physical therapy, vocational training, and special training such as speech therapy.

Rheumatologist: A specialist in the non-surgical treatment of rheumatic illnesses, especially arthritis.

Saddle Embolus A large blood clot that straddles the arterial bifurcation and
blocks both branches causing death.

Saline Solution: Salt solution, often adjusted to the normal salinity of the human body. Salt, in medicine, is referring to sodium chloride. Sodium chloride is common table salt and the salt concentrated in the earth and in seawater.

Scarlet Fever: An infectious bacterial disease affecting especially children, and causing fever and a scarlet rash. It is caused by streptococci and was often deadly before penicillin was discovered.

Self-limited disease: A condition that resolves spontaneously with or without specific treatment, such as the common cold.

Septic shock: A medical condition resulting from a severe infection and sepsis, though the microbe may be systemic or localized to a particular site. It can cause multiple organ dysfunction syndrome (formerly known as multiple organ failure) and death.

Sex Hormones: Hormones — estrogen, progesterone and testosterone — affecting sexual development, general metabolic functions and reproduction.

Shingles vaccine: Specifically designed to protect people against Herpes virus that causes shingles only. Will not protect people against other forms of herpes, such as genital herpes.

Small Pox: An acute infectious disease caused by a virus and now almost completely eradicated. Smallpox was characterized by high fever and large sores on the body that leave scars.

Sociologists: Study the organization, institutions, and development of societies, with a particular interest in identifying causes of the changing relationships among individuals and groups.

Specialization: Breaking down of people into individual body parts.

Stage IV breast cancer: Cancer that has spread to other areas of the body, such as the brain, bones, lung and liver.

Statins: Any of a group of drugs that act to reduce levels of fats, including triglycerides and cholesterol, in the blood.

Statistic: A fact or piece of data from a study of a large quantity of numerical data.

Subdural Hematoma: A collection of blood outside the brain. Subdural hematomas are usually caused by severe head injuries. The bleeding and increased pressure on the brain from a subdural hematoma can be life threatening.

Subspecialty: A narrow field of study or work within a specialty. Example: pediatric dermatology, cardiology or gastroenterology in internal medicine, geriatric psychiatry, thoracic surgery, hematology, oncology, etc.

Surgical Intensive Care Unit: Hospital unit designated for care of critically ill surgical patients.

Terminal patient: Patient suffering with a disease that cannot be cured or adequately treated and that is reasonably expected to result in the death of the patient within a short period of time.

Testosterone: The "male hormone" — a sex hormone produced by the testes that encourages the development of male sexual characteristics, stimulates the activity of the male secondary sex characteristics.

Thyphus: an infectious disease caused by rickettsiae, characterized by a purple rash, headaches, fever, and usually delirium, and historically a cause of high mortality during wars and famines. There are several forms, transmitted by vectors such as lice, ticks, mites, and rat fleas.

Tuberculosis bacilli: Widespread, and in many cases fatal, infectious disease caused by various strains of mycobacteria, usually Mycobacterium tuberculosis.

Tumor: Swelling of a part of the body, generally without inflammation, caused by an abnormal growth of tissue — benign or malignant.

Ulcer: Open sore on an external or internal surface of the body, caused by a break in the skin or mucous membrane that fails to heal.

Ultrafast CT Scan Electron Beam Computerized Tomography (EBCT): Noninvasive test for the detection of coronary artery disease (CAD). Ultrafast computerized tomography is designed to measure calcium deposits in the coronary arteries.

Upper Endoscopy: A procedure that involves placing a tube with a camera at its end into the stomach to evaluate the lining of the esophagus and stomach and to take samples—biopsies—of the stomach, esophagus and culture the contents for bacteria—where and when necessary. (Also known as a gastroscopy).

Urethra: The duct by which urine is conveyed out of the body from the bladder.

Urinary Tract Infections UTI: An infection in any part of urinary system — kidneys, ureters, bladder and urethra. Most commonly the infections involve the lower urinary tract — the bladder and the urethra.

Urologist: Physician who specializes in diseases of the urinary organs in females and the urinary and sex organs in males.

Uterine wall: Entire thickness of the womb. Muscle and uterine lining.

Yeast Infections: Infection of the vagina caused by a fungus known as Candida. A vaginal yeast infection is characterized by itching, burning, soreness, pain during intercourse and/or urination, and vaginal discharge that is typically cheesy white in color.

RECOMMENDATIONS FOR FURTHER READING

1. John Abramson, MD. *Overdosed America: The Broken Promise of American Medicine,* Harper Perennial, 3rd Edition. March 5, 2013.

2. Mehmet C. Oz, MD and Michael F. Roizen MD. *YOU: The Owner's Manual: An Insider's Guide to the Body That Will Make You Healthier and Younger.* William Morrow Paperback: Updated, Expand edition. December 17, 2013.

3. Michael Roizen, MD. *This Is Your Do-over: The 7 Secrets of Losing Weight, Living Longer, and Getting a Second Chance at the Life You Want.* Scribner. February 24, 2015.

4. Mehmet C. Oz, MD. *Healing from the Heart: How Unconventional Wisdom Unleashes the Power of Modern Medicine.* Plume. 1st Edition. October 1, 1999.

5. Mehmet C. Oz, MD and Michael F. Roizen, MD. *YOU: The Smart Patient: An Insider's Handbook for Getting the Best Treatment.* Scribner. 1st Edition. February 10, 2006.

6. James Thomas Williams. *The Patient Advocate's Handbook: 300 Questions And Answers To Help You Care For Your Loved One At The Hospital And At Home.* Panglossian Press. January 1, 2010.

7. Bruce Jansson. *Improving Healthcare Through Advocacy: A Guide for the Health and Helping Professions.* Wiley. 1st Edition. January 25, 2011.

8. Staff of the *Dallas Morning News. First Do No Harm: Patient safety crisis at one of America's landmark public hospitals.* The Dallas Morning News. 1st Edition. November 28, 2012.

9. Marty Makary. *Unaccountable: What Hospitals Won't Tell You and How Transparency Can Revolutionize Health Care.* Bloomsbury Press. Reprint Edition. October 15, 2013.

10. Atul Gawande. *Being Mortal: Medicine and What Matters in the End.* Metropolitan Books. 1st Edition. October 7, 2014.

11. Atul Gawande. *The Checklist Manifesto: How to Get Things Right.* Picado. Reprint Edition. January 4, 2011.

12. Otis Webb Brawley and Paul Goldberg. *How We Do Harm: A Doctor Breaks Ranks About Being Sick in America.* St. Martin's Griffin. Reprint Edition. October 30, 2012.

13. Leana Wen, MD and Joshua Kosowsky, MD. *When Doctors Don't Listen: How to Avoid Misdiagnoses and Unnecessary Tests.* St. Martin's Griffin. Reprint Edition. June 24, 2014.

14. Barry Werth. *The Antidote: Inside the World of New Pharma.* Simon & Schuster. Reprint edition. February 4, 2014.

15. Peter Gotzsche. *Deadly Medicines and Organised Crime: How Big Pharma Has Corrupted Healthcare.* Radcliffe Medical Press LTD. 1st Edition. August 31, 2013.

16. Ben Goldacre. *Bad Pharma: How Drug Companies Mislead Doctors and Harm Patients.* Faber & Faber. Reprint Edition. February 5, 2013.

17. Betsy McCaughey. *Unnecessary Deaths: The Human and Financial Costs of Hospital Infections.* Committee to Reduce Infection Deaths (RID). 2005.

HELPFUL ORGANIZATIONS:

Patient Voice Institute
www.gopvi.org
patientvoiceinstitute.org

CarePartner
www.carepartner.com

Alliance of Professional Health Advocates (APHA)
http://www.aphadvocates.org

Insurance Fraud
www.insurancefraud.org

AARP Foundation
www.aarp.org/Foundation

BHI Online
http://www.bhionline.org

Hospital Infections
www.hospitalinfection.org

REFERENCES AND ENDNOTES:

1   Jewell, Kevin and Lisa McGiffert. "To Err is Human—To Delay is Deadly." Consumers Union. May 2009. <http://safepatientproject. org/pdf/safepatientproject.org-to_delay_is_deadly-2009_05.pdf>.

2   James, JT. "A New Evidence-Based Estimate of Patient Harms Associated With Hospital Care." *Journal of Patient Safety.* 2013. Volume 9, Issue 3, 122-128.

3   Petersen, Melody. "A Veil Of Secrecy Shields Hospitals Where Outbreaks Occur." *Los Angeles Times*, Apr. 18, 2015.

4   Baker, SL. "Johns Hopkins Researcher Speaks Out: Arrogance Of Doctors Is Killing Tens Of Thousands Of Patients." *Natural News.* Aug. 3, 2010. <http://www.naturalnews.com/029350_doctors_patients.html >.

5   Bell, SK, AA White, JP Yi-Frazier, and TH Gallagher. "Transparency When Things Go Wrong: Physician Attitudes About Report-

ing Medical Errors to Patients, Peers, and Institutions." *Journal of Patient Safety*. Feb. 24, 2015.

6   Britta, A, PG Stumpf, and J Schulkin, "Medical Error Reporting, Patient Safety and the Physician." *Journal of Patient Safety*. Sep. 2009; 5(3):176-9. Doi: 10.1097/PTS.0b013e3181b320b0.

7   James, JT. "A New Evidence-Based Estimate of Patient Harms Associated with Hospital Care." *Journal of Patient Safety*. 2013. Volume 9, Issue 3, 122-128.

8   "U.S. Medical School Applications and Matriculants by School, State of Legal Residence, and Sex," Association of American Medical Colleges. 2014. <https://www.aamc.org/download/321442/data/factstable1.pdf>.

9   Miller, M, KR Mcgowen, and JH Quillen. "The Painful Truth: Physicians Are Not Invincible." *South Med J*. 2000. 93 (10).

10   Wible, Pamela. "When Doctors Commit Suicide, It's Often Hushed Up." *The Washington Post*. July 14, 2014. <http://www.washingtonpost.com/national/health-science/when-doctors-commit-suicide-its-often-hushed-up/2014/07/14/d8f6eda8-e0fb-11e3-9743-bb9b59cde7b9_story.html>.

11   Kao, H, R Conant, T Soriano, and W McCormick. "The Past, Present, and Future of House Calls." Clinics in Geriatric Medicine. Feb. 2009. (1):19-34. Doi: 10.1016/j.cger.2008.10.005.

12   Stuck, AE, M. Egger, A. Hammer, CW Minder, and JC Beck. "Home Visits to Prevent Nursing Home Admission and Functional

Decline in Elderly People: Systematic Review and Meta-regression Analysis." *Journal of the American Medical Association*. 2002; 287(8): 1022-1028. Doi: 10.1001/jama.287.8.1022. <http://jama. jamanetwork.com/article.aspx?articleid=194675>.

[13] Span, P. "No Place Like Home." *New York Times*. June 20, 2010. <http://newoldage.blogs.nytimes.com/2010/06/30/no-place-like-home>.

[14] Kao, H., R. Conant, T. Soriano, and W. McCormick. "The Past, Present, and Future of House Calls." Clinics in Geriatric Medicine. Feb. 2009. (1):19-34. Doi: 10.1016/j.cger.2008.10.005.

[15] Mishori, R. "House Calls Making A Comeback." *The Washington Post*. Mar. 24, 2009. <http://www.washingtonpost.com/wpdyn/content/article/2009/03/23/AR2009032301745.html>.

[16] Sivastraba. "Is Medicine A Cult?" The Student Doctor Network, General Residential Issues. Mar. 29, 2006. SDN – Student Doctor Network Web Forum. <http://forums.studentdoctor.net/threads/is-medicine-a-cult.269745/>.

[17] A: Hall, Harriet, "Re-thinking the Annual Physical." Science-Based Medicine. Feb. 21, 2012. <https://www.sciencebasedmedicine.org/re-thinking-the-annual-physical/>.
B: Emanuel, Ezekiel J. "Skip Your Annual Physical." *The New York Times*. Jan. 8, 2015. <http://www.nytimes.com/2015/01/09/opinion/skip-your-annual-physical.html?_r=0>.
C: CBS News. "Do you really need a yearly physical exam?" CBS interactive. Jan. 12, 2015. <http://www.cbsnews.com/news/do-you-really-need-a-yearly-physical-exam>.

18 "Putting Patients First: Patient-Centered Collaborative Care, A Discussion Paper." Canadian Medical Association, July 2007. <http://fhs.mcmaster.ca/surgery/documents/Collaborative CareBackgrounderRevised.pdf>.

19 Abramson, J. *Overdosed America: The Broken Promise of American Medicine*, Harper Perennial, 3rd Edition. Mar. 5, 2013.

20 "Health At a Glance – OECD Indicators." OECD. Nov. 2013. <http://www.oecd.org/els/health-systems/Health-at-a-Glance-2013-Chart-set.pdf>.

21 Ingraham, C. "Our Infant Mortality Rate Is a National Embarrassment." *The Washington Post*. Sept. 29, 2014. <http://www. washingtonpost.com/blogs/wonkblog/wp/2014/09/29/our-infant-mortality-rate-is-a-national-embarrassment/>.

22 Ng, M., T. Fleming, M. Robinson, et al. "Global, Regional and National Prevalence of Overweight and Obesity In Children and Adults During 1980–2013: A Systematic Analysis For The Global Burden of Disease Study 2013." Aug. 30, 2014, 384 (9945): 766-81. Doi: 10.1016/S0140-6736 (14)60460-8. Epub. May 29, 2014.

23 "US Has World's 7th Highest Cancer Rate: AICR Experts Highlight Role of Diet, Weight, Physical Activity on Cancer Incidence." American Institute for Cancer Research. Jan. 24, 2011.

24 Pasternak, S. "End-Of-Life Care Constitues Third Rail Of U.S. Health Care Policy Debate," The Medicare NewsGroup, June 3, 2013, 16:03.

25 "US Health System Ranks Last Among Eleven Countries On Measures of Access, Equity, Quality, Efficiency, And Healthy Lives." The Commonwealth Fund. June 16, 2014. <http://www.commonwealthfund.org/publications/press-releases/2014/jun/us-health-system-ranks-last>.

26 Abramson, J. *Overdosed America: The Broken Promise of American Medicine*, Harper Perennial, 3rd Edition. Mar. 5, 2013.

27 "OTC Sales by Category 2011-2014." Consumer Healthcare Products Association. <http://www.chpa.org/OTCsCategory.aspx>.

28 Bronnenberg, B, JP Dubé, M Gentzkow, and JM Shapiro. "Do Pharmacists Buy Bayer? Informed Shoppers and the Brand Premium." Jan. 2015. <http://www.brown.edu/Research/Shapiro/pdfs/generics.pdf>.

29 Johnson, B. "100 Leading National Advertisers." June 20, 2011. http://adage.com/article/news/ad-spending-100-leading-national-advertisers/228267/.

30 Healthcare and Pharma. "6 CVS Leads Pharmacy Chains Opening Walk-In Clinics - Drugstores Are Shaking Up The Traditional Path To Care." EMarketer. July 15, 2014. <http://www.emarketer.com/Article/CVS-Leads-Pharmacy-Chains-Opening-Walk-In-Clinics/1011468>.

31 Gunderman, R. "The Case Against Drugstore Clinics." *The Atlantic*. Oct. 11, 2014. <http://www.theatlantic.com/health/archive/2014/10/the-case-against-drugstore-clinics/381023/>.

[32] Nisen, M. "The American Health Care System Should Be Terrified of the Rise of the Pharmacy Clinic." *Business Insider*. July 11, 2013. <http://www.businessinsider.com/the-rise-of-the-pharmacy-clinic-2013-7>.

[33] Hagopian, J. "The Evils Of Big Pharma Exposed." *GlobalResearch*. Jan. 18, 2015. <http://www.globalresearch.ca/the-evils-of-big-pharma-exposed/5425382>.

[34] Ventola, CL. "Direct to Consumer Pharmaceutical Advertising: Therapeutic or Toxic?" P&T Volume 36. Oct. 2011. No. 10. Pp. 669-672.

[35] Ventola, CL. "Direct to Consumer Pharmaceutical Advertising: Therapeutic or Toxic?" P&T Volume 36. Oct. 2011. No. 10. Pp. 669-672.

[36] Connors, AL. "Big Bad Pharma: An Ethical Analysis of Physician-Directed and Consumer-Directed Marketing Tactics." *Albany Law Review*. 2009. 73 (1) 243-282.

[37] Frosch, DL, P Krueger, et al. "Creating Demand for Prescription Drugs: A Content Analysis of Television Direct-to-Consumer Advertising." *Annals of Family Medicine*. 2007; 5 (1) 179.

[38] Frosch, DL, D Grande, DM Tarn, and RL Kravitz. "A decade of controversy: balancing policy with evidence in the regulation of prescription drug advertising." *American Journal of Public Health*. 2010: 100 (1) 24-32. Doi: 10.2105/AJPH.2008.153767.

[39] Delbaere, M, MC Smith. "Health Care Knowledge and Consumer Learning: The Case of Direct to Consumer Advertising." Health Mark Q. 2009; 23 (3) 9-29.

[40] Connors, AL. Big Bad Pharma: An ethical analysis of physician-directed and consumer-directed marketing tactics. *Albany Law Review*. 2009; 73 (1) 243-282.

[41] Abramson, J. *Overdosed America: The Broken Promise of American Medicine*, Harper Perennial, 3rd Edition. Mar. 5, 2013.

[42] Presley, H. "Vioxx and The Merck Team Effort." Duke Ethics. The Keenan Institute For Ethics. 2009. <http://kenan.ethics.duke.edu/wp-content/uploads/2012/08/Vioxx_FinalDesignedCase2015.pdf>.

[43] Elliot, S. "DDB Worldwide Wins Merck Account." *The New York Times*. Feb. 20, 2001. http://www.nytimes.com/2001/02/20/business/the-media-business-advertising-addenda-ddb-worldwide-wins-merck-account.html.

[44] Ventola, CL. "Direct to Consumer Pharmaceutical Advertising: Therapeutic or Toxic?" P&T Volume 36. Oct. 2011. No. 10. Pp. 669 – 684.

[45] Abramson, J. *Overdosed America: The Broken Promise of American Medicine*, Harper Perennial, 3rd Edition. Mar. 5, 2013. Pp. 23-38.

[46] Mercola, J. "The 6 Types of Pills Big Pharma Wants You Hooked On for Life." Mercola.com. May 14, 2012. <http://articles.mercola.

com/sites/articles/archive/2012/05/14/mercks-adhd-drugs-unsafe.aspx>.

47   Abramson, J. *Overdosed America: The Broken Promise of American Medicine*, Harper Perennial, 3rd Edition. Mar. 5, 2013. Pp. 807.

48   Lal, R. "Patent And Exclusivity." FDA/CDER SBIA Chronicles. May 19, 2015. <http://www.fda.gov/downloads/Drugs/ DevelopmentApprovalProcess/SmallBusinessAssistance/ UCM447307.pdf>

49   James, JT. "A New Evidence-Based Estimate of Patient Harms Associated With Hospital Care." *Journal of Patient Safety*. 2013. Volume 9, Issue 3. Pp. 122-128.

50   Institute of Medicine. "To Err is Human: Building a Safer Health System." National Academy of Sciences. Nov. 1999.

51   Rauch, J. "The Hospital is No Place for the Elderly." *Atlantic Magazine*. Dec. 2013. <http://www.theatlantic.com/magazine/ archive/2013/12/the-home-remedy-for-old-age/354680/>.

52   Creditor, M. "Hazards of Hospitalization of the Elderly." *Annals of Internal Medicine*. Feb. 1, 1993. Vol. 118, Issue 3. Pp. 219-223.

53   Hoenig, HM and LZ Rubenstein, "Hospital-associated deconditioning and dysfunction." (Editorial) Journal of the American Geriatrics Society. 1991. 39: 220-2.

54   Davis, R. "The Doctor Who Championed Hand-Washing and Briefly Saved Lives." NPR. Jan. 12, 2015. <http://www.npr.org/

sections/health-shots/2015/01/12/375663920/the-doctor-who-championed-hand-washing-and-saved-women-s-lives>.

55   Petersen, M. "A veil of secrecy shields hospitals where outbreaks occur." *Los Angeles Times*. Apr. 18, 2015. <http://www.latimes.com/business/la-fi-hospital-outbreaks-secrecy-20150419-story.html>.

56   Sanghavi, Darshak. "How to Sell Germ Warfare: Can hand sanitizers like Purell really stop people from getting the flu?" *Slate Online*. Feb. 4, 2010. <http://www.slate.com/articles/news_and_politics/prescriptions/2010/02/how_to_sell_germ_warfare.html>.

57   Svetla Slavova, PhD, Terry L. Bunn, PhD, and Jeffery Talbert, PhD. "Drug Overdose Surveillance Using Hospital Discharge Data." Public Health Reports. Sept–Oct. 2014. Vol. 129. Pp. 437-449.

58   Makary, M. *Unaccountable: What Hospitals Won't Tell You and How Transparency Can Revolutionize Health Care*. Bloomsbury Press. Sept. 18, 2012. Pp. 106.

59   Tai-Seale, M, T McGuire, and W Zhang. "Time Allocation in Primary Care Office Visits." Oct. 2007. 42(5): 1871–1894. Doi: 10.1111/J: 1457-6773.2006.00689.x

60   Campion, R. *The Invisible Worm*. New York: Macmillan. 1972.

ABOUT THE AUTHORS

DR. ERIKA SCHWARTZ

Erika Schwartz, M.D., is the founder of Evolved Science (E/S), a personalized medicine practice with headquarters in New York City. Dr. Schwartz specializes in wellness and disease prevention through the use of conventional, integrative and lifestyle medicine. She is a fierce patient advocate who teaches doctors and medical students how to develop close and responsible relationships with their patients. She is the author of four books and an international health thought leader. She has made numerous media appearances on PBS, *The View*, *Good Morning America*, *Good Day New York*, and many other TV and radio programs. She is a sought after speaker and writer, having been quoted in and written for the *Wall Street Journal*, *New York Times*, *Daily Mail*, *Vogue* and many others.

MELISSA JO PELTIER

Co-author of five *New York Times* Bestsellers with TV's Dog Whisperer, Cesar Millan, as well as *The Mommy Docs Ultimate Guide to Pregnancy and Birth*, Ms. Peltier is also a two-time Emmy-award winning writer, producer and director who has accumulated more than fifty national and international film and TV awards and accolades, including a Humanitas and Peabody Award and four nominations from the Writer's Guild of America. Her first novel *Reality Boulevard* (Apostrophe Books Ltd, UK) was named by Kirkus Reviews as one of its "Best Indies" for 2013. She is a Boston native who survived twenty years in L.A. and now lives happily and healthily in New York with her husband, film and television writer/director John Gray.